DO YOU KNOW THE ANSWERS TO THESE LIFE-OR-DEATH QUESTIONS?

What are the symptoms of high blood pressure?

What organs can be irreparably damaged if high blood pressure goes undetected?

Does too much salt cause high blood pressure?

Can licorice or tobacco cause high blood pressure?

Should pregnant women have special concerns about high blood pressure?

What is the connection between being overweight and having high blood pressure?

What can make you a likely candidate for high blood pressure?

What is the dangerous "bounce back" effect of suddenly stopping medication?

YOU'LL FIND THE ANSWERS TO THESE AND MANY OF YOUR QUESTIONS IN... HIGH BLOOD PRESSURE

HIGH
BLOOD
PRESSURE

Neil B. Shulman

Associate Professor
of Medicine
Department of
Medicine
Emory University
School of Medicine
and Grady Memorial
Hospital
Atlanta, Georgia

Elijah Saunders

Associate Professor
of Medicine
Department of
Medicine
Chief, Division of
Hypertension
Clinical Director,
Center for Vascular
Biology and
Hypertension
University of
Maryland School of
Medicine and
Hospital
Baltimore, Maryland

W. Dallas Hall

Professor of
Medicine
Department of
Medicine
Director, Division of
Hypertension
Director, General
Clinical Research
Center
Emory University
School of Medicine,
Grady Memorial
Hospital
and Emory Hospital
Atlanta, Georgia

Illustrations by Scott Thorn Barrows, A.M.I.
Clinical Assistant Professor
University of Illinois Medical Center

A DELL BOOK

*This book is dedicated to all of our
patients. You have been an inspiration
to help us learn about high blood
pressure and how to treat it.*

Published by
Dell Publishing
a division of Bantam Doubleday Dell Publishing Group, Inc.
1540 Broadway
New York, New York 10036

ISBN: 0-440-21693-1

Reprinted by arrangement with
Macmillan Publishing Company
Printed in the United States of America
Published simultaneously in Canada

First Dell Printing: October 1989
Revised edition: January 1993

10   9   8   7   6

RAD

Contents

ACKNOWLEDGMENTS

Our appreciation to friends and colleagues
who have helped with this book:

Sally Graver
Marlis McDowell Jackson
Eleanora Morton
Charlene Shucker

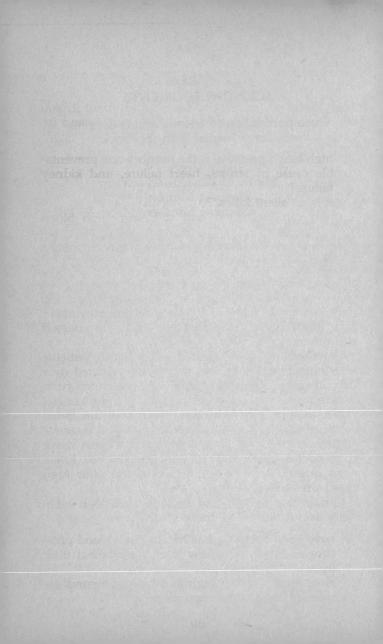

TO THE READER

High blood pressure—you have heard about it, you may even have it, but do you really understand it? Do you realize that...

- high blood pressure is the number-one preventable cause of stroke, heart failure, and kidney failure?
- it is a "silent killer"?
- you can feel great and still have high blood pressure?
- treatment is fairly simple and can prevent almost all of the problems?

The purpose of this book is to present in accessible, easy-to-read language the newest therapies and the most important things you need to know about high blood pressure so that you can help yourself and others.

Together, we have treated over **20,000** patients with high blood pressure; we have conducted over **fifty** high-blood-pressure research trials; we have lectured to doctors, nurses, patients and the general public around the world. And now, with this book, we want to give you an objective, practical resource to answer your questions, to expand upon what your doctor has told you, and to help you know what questions you need to ask about your high blood pressure.

Certain people will find parts of this book especially useful, including those who...

- have been diagnosed as having high blood pressure and want to know how it will affect their lives.
- have relatives with high blood pressure and are worried about their own risks.

- want to understand how blood pressure is measured.
- want to know more about special tests their doctor has ordered to evaluate their high blood pressure.
- do not realize that although muscle weakness, impotence, loss of sexual desire, fatigue, depression, and other problems might be caused by blood pressure drugs, these side effects are often avoidable.
- need to understand that stopping their medication, even when they are feeling good, can be dangerous.
- do not fully appreciate the importance of controlling their blood pressure.

Like your doctor, who is your most important resource, the three of us want you to have your blood pressure controlled without problems. We hope this book will help you.

W. Dallas Hall, M.D.   *Elijah Saunders, M.D.*
Neil B. Shulman, M.D.

1

What Is High Blood Pressure and How Do You Get It?

THE SILENT KILLER

High blood pressure is unlike any other disease. It is potentially extremely serious, but usually does not affect how you feel day to day. It is often referred to as "the silent killer" because there are few symptoms in the early stages of the disease. People with high blood pressure often do not even know or suspect they have it unless their blood pressure has been measured. So they go along, never realizing that this condition may be slowly causing serious damage to the eyes and kidneys and putting them at risk of stroke, kidney disease, and heart disease, including sudden death.

Hundreds of millions of people in the world suffer from high blood pressure; in the United States alone, at least 50 million Americans have or are at risk of the consequences of high blood pressure. About 65 percent of people with high blood pressure are aware that they have it, yet fewer than half of them are being treated. Of those who are being treated, only 21 percent have their blood pressure controlled to a level of 140/90 mm Hg or less. This low control rate is the result of people not understanding the seriousness of the problem, not taking the prescribed medications correctly, not making necessary changes in lifestyle, or not seeing the doctor on a regular basis.

When the patient does get treatment, in the great majority of cases, high blood pressure can be controlled and serious damage avoided.

HIGH BLOOD PRESSURE

High blood pressure (HBP) is also called hypertension. "Blood pressure" is the force with which your heart pumps blood through the body. Occasional increases in blood pressure levels are not unusual. For example, if you shovel snow, run to catch a bus, carry a suitcase, or unload heavy groceries, your heart beats faster and more powerfully, raising your blood pressure as it works to meet the added demands of strenuous activity. If you are angry or excited, your nerves send out signals to stimulate your heart and narrow your blood vessels, and both of these results will, in turn, act to increase your blood pressure. However, if your blood pressure reaches abnormally high levels and stays high, then you are considered to have high blood pressure.

ESSENTIAL HYPERTENSION

High blood pressure is known to physicians as "essential hypertension." This can be a misleading term because the condition is neither necessary (essential) nor a condition of high nervous tension (hypertension). In medical terminology, however, essential hypertension refers to high blood pressure that is the result of unknown or undetected causes. It is sometimes called "primary" hypertension (see *Glossary*).

If you have high blood pressure, you probably have essential hypertension, which accounts for 90 to 95 percent of all cases. There is a much smaller chance that you may suffer from the other major class of high blood pressure, "secondary" hypertension, which has some identifiable causes and often can be cured by surgery.

CAUSES OF HIGH BLOOD PRESSURE

Although we do not know the exact cause or causes for most cases of high blood pressure, we find that certain risk factors or associations usually are present. These include ethnicity, age, where you live, salt intake, weight, stress, alcohol consumption, lack of exercise, and heredity.

Ethnicity

For many years, physicians have recognized that high blood pressure occurs one-and-a-half to two times more frequently among blacks than among whites. It develops, on the average, five to ten years earlier; is generally more severe, with higher blood pressure levels; and progresses more rapidly with earlier complications. The racial difference in blood pressure may appear as early as the late teenage years. This greater frequency of high blood pressure among black families may be influenced by environmental factors. However, when blacks migrate from the South and southeastern parts of the United States, they still have hypertension more frequently than whites. It should be emphasized that there are many things that all ethnic groups can do to control high blood pressure even though they may be predisposed to it. Chapter 9 emphasizes what you can do to help control your blood pressure.

Age

A newborn baby's blood pressure is relatively low. Generally speaking, blood pressure goes up naturally as you get older. There are normal limits for blood pressure for children, teenagers, and adults. If the rise is too sudden or too great, then you have high blood pressure.

Environmental Factors

Although hereditary factors clearly play a major role in causing high blood pressure, they do not explain why many people develop this problem when their relatives did not. This suggests that, in many cases, your environment and lifestyle may determine whether you develop high blood pressure. Environmental and lifestyle factors include where you live, salt intake, weight, stress, alcohol consumption, lack of exercise, exposure to certain chemicals in the work place, birth control pills in some cases, many addictive drugs, interaction with other medications (prescription or over-the-counter), and many other less proven factors.

Where You Live. You are most likely to develop hypertension if you live in certain parts of the world, such as the southeastern regions of the United States. The reasons for this are not clear. Also, within certain regions of the country, if you live in the inner city, especially if you are black and poor, you are more likely to have high blood pressure than if you live in the suburbs.

Salt and Other Chemicals. It has often been said, "You are what you eat." In fact, high salt (sodium) intake does seem to relate to an increased likelihood of having high blood pressure. Worldwide population studies have shown, for example, that the frequency of strokes, which are mostly caused by high blood pressure, is the highest among people who have a high level of salt in their diet, such as the Japanese. Conversely, people such as the Solomon Islanders of the South Pacific and those living in rural areas in Africa, who consume little salt, have very low rates of high blood pressure.

Animal studies also support the connection between salt intake and blood pressure. Researchers have found that certain strains of rats, if fed a high-salt diet, develop high blood pressure very rapidly.

Recent studies suggest that some people who have or are at risk of getting high blood pressure are not harmed by a high salt intake; they are not "salt sensitive." But most hypertensive patients are salt sensitive; they will develop higher blood pressure by eating too much salt. Blacks are among those hypertensives who are usually salt sensitive and for whom a low-salt diet is recommended, both for treatment and prevention of high blood pressure.

If you do not have enough potassium in your diet, you are more likely to develop hypertension, especially if you eat a lot of salt. Recent studies also suggest that certain patients may have high blood pressure if they do not get enough calcium.

Weight. Excessive weight is often associated with increased blood pressure. This does not mean that if you are lean and thin you will not get high blood pressure, but simply that if you are overweight, or gain too much weight, you are two to six times more likely to develop this condition.

Stress. Stress produced by various circumstances can make you more likely to develop high blood pressure. It also makes treatment more difficult. A few studies have suggested that people in certain high-stress occupations and those whose jobs involve heavy physical labor are more likely to have high blood pressure.

Stress produced by poverty, crowding, racial tension, and low socioeconomic and educational status also contributes to high blood pressure. This may help explain some of the unusually high rates of hypertension among blacks in the United States. Studies have also suggested that skin color may be related to high blood pressure. More darker-skinned blacks have hypertension than do those with lighter complexions. Social scientists have raised the question of whether skin color may heavily influence how blacks are treated in their environment; that is, whether darker-skinned individuals experience greater social, occupational, and economic stresses, which are all related to high blood pressure.

Alcohol. Alcohol can also contribute to high blood pressure. Studies show that heavy drinkers of alcohol have higher rates of high blood pressure than do people who drink less. Drug therapy is less effective in patients who drink heavily. Blood pressure levels can often improve when patients stop drinking.

Lack of Exercise. An inactive lifestyle can lead to high blood pressure, whether the condition runs in your family or not. In addition, if you do not get much exercise, you tend to become overweight, which further contributes to high blood pressure. Conversely, it appears that if you increase your physical activity and get regular exercise, you may help to reduce your blood pressure and perhaps delay the onset of hypertension.

Hereditary Factors

High blood pressure tends to run in families. If your mother and father both have high blood pressure or a complication of high blood pressure (stroke, heart attack, kidney failure, etc.) there is a strong possibility that you will also develop high blood pressure at some point in your life, and it is likely to appear about ten years earlier than it might if your parents did not have this disorder.

In general, blood relatives of hypertensive individuals develop high blood pressure more frequently than do relatives of nonhypertensive individuals. This suggests that some inherited factor predisposes certain people to developing this disease. The strongest research evidence supporting this theory comes from studies of twins.

Among fraternal twins (produced from two eggs), if one has high blood pressure, there is a strong likelihood that the other will also develop high blood pressure at some time in life, even if the twins do not grow up in the same environment. Among twins that are identical (produced from one egg), if one has high blood pressure, the other is almost certain to have it as well, even if they do not grow up in the same environment.

2

How Is Blood Pressure Measured?

SYSTOLE AND DIASTOLE

Your blood pressure varies with the beat of your heart. Figure 1 illustrates how this happens. Every time the main chamber of the heart squeezes (systole), blood spurts into the large arteries, stretching their elastic walls. When the heart chamber relaxes (diastole), the arterial walls spring back, keeping the blood flowing between heartbeats. The high pressure generated by the squeezing of the chambers (ventricles) is called the "systolic" pressure. The lower pressure generated while the heart relaxes is known as the "diastolic" pressure.

Blood pressure measurements are written as two numbers. For example, 120/80—with the systolic level on the top and the diastolic level on the bottom.

UNITS OF MEASUREMENT

The units of blood pressure measurement are millimeters (mm) of mercury (Hg). Thus, a systolic blood pressure of 140 mm Hg means that the pressure in the artery is enough to raise a narrow column of liquid mercury 140 millimeters, or about 5.5 inches. Mercury is used instead of water because it is about thirteen times heavier, and shorter tubes can be used for the measurement. (A systolic blood pressure of 140 mm Hg would raise a similar column of water almost 6 feet high).

WHAT THE NUMBERS MEAN

Normal Blood Pressure

In most adults, blood pressure is considered to be normal when the top number (systolic) is less than 140 mm Hg and the bottom number (diastolic) is less than 90. These values assume that the measurement is made properly, using the correct size blood pressure cuff when you are sitting and relaxed. Both the top and bottom numbers usually vary by at least 20 mm Hg at different times during the day. The top number (systolic), for example, normally increases to over 160 mm Hg with exercise and may fall to less than 100 mm Hg during sleep. Blood pressure is usually highest in the early morning and is typically lower in the evening, especially while you sleep.

Not a lot of information can be gained from a single elevated blood pressure reading. That is why

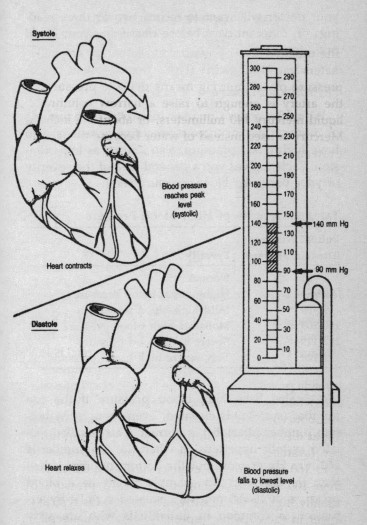

Figure 1 SYSTOLIC AND DIASTOLIC PRESSURE

your doctor will want to record two or three readings on different days before classifying your blood pressure.

High Blood Pressure

When the bottom number (diastolic) is 90 mm Hg or more on two or three consecutive occasions, you have high blood pressure, also known as hypertension. Table 1 gives you a general idea of the severity of your particular blood pressure level.

TABLE 1. Severity of High Blood Pressure

Bottom Number (Diastolic pressure)	Severity
<85	Normal
85-89	High-normal blood pressure
90-99	Mild high blood pressure
100-109	Moderate high blood pressure
110-119	Severe high blood pressure
≥120	Very severe high blood pressure

You also have high blood pressure if the top number (systolic) is elevated, even though the bottom number (diastolic) is normal. This is called isolated systolic hypertension when the top number is 160 mm Hg or more but the bottom number is less than 90 mm Hg. An example might be a blood pressure of 190/80 mm Hg. Isolated systolic hypertension is common in individuals who are sixty years of age or older. It is also common in patients with diabetes.

Knowing your blood pressure numbers allows you to keep track of your progress if you are on a special diet or if you are taking blood pressure medicines. The "goal" of most treatment programs is to gradually reduce the bottom number (or diastolic pressure) to below 90 mm Hg and often also the top number (or systolic pressure) to below 160 mm Hg. Regular blood pressure measurements enable your doctor to monitor your progress and treatment.

BLOOD PRESSURE EQUIPMENT AND HOW IT WORKS

The measurement of blood pressure requires two pieces of equipment: an arm cuff that has a pressure gauge attached to it, and a listening device. The cuff and pressure gauge are called a sphygmomanometer and the listening device is called a stethoscope.

Figure 2 shows how the cuff works. When it is wrapped around the upper arm and inflated, the air pressure in the cuff pushes the main artery of the arm (brachial artery) against the nearby bone (humerus). When the pressure in the cuff is equal to or greater than the pressure in the artery, it stops the flow of blood through the artery, and the pulse on the thumb side of your wrist (the radial artery) disappears.

Reducing the cuff pressure allows the blood to flow again. The stethoscope is placed directly over the artery to hear the tapping or knocking sounds made by the flow of blood through the compressed artery. The pressure when the very

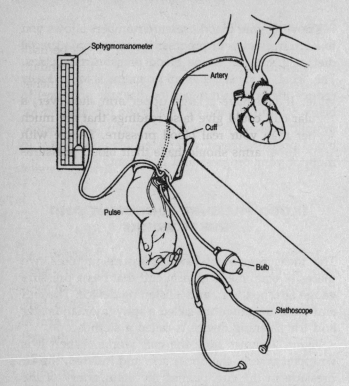

Sphygmomanometer

Artery

Cuff

Pulse

Bulb

Stethoscope

Figure 2 BLOOD PRESSURE MEASUREMENT EQUIPMENT

first sound can be heard is the systolic blood pressure.

As pressure in the cuff continues to be released, tapping and swishing sounds can be heard as the blood flows through the compressed artery. Finally all sounds disappear when the cuff pressure has been reduced to a point equal to or less than the diastolic blood pressure when the heart is relaxed.

Large and Small Cuffs

The proper size blood pressure cuff must be used to measure blood pressure correctly. The standard blood pressure cuff used for adults is 4.75 to 5 inches wide. If you have a large upper arm, however, a regular cuff could give false readings that are much higher than your real blood pressure. People with large upper arms should have their blood pressures measured with a larger-size cuff. This is usually called an "adult obese" or "obese" arm cuff and is 6 to 6.25 inches wide.

How can you tell if you need to use the larger-size cuff? First, take a tape measure and measure the distance from your elbow along the outside of your arm to the outermost top bone of your shoulder. Divide this by two to find the middle of your upper arm. Lightly mark this point with a ballpoint pen. Now place the tape around your arm at this point and measure the size of this middle part of your upper arm. If it is more than 13 inches, then your blood pressure measurements probably should be made with a larger cuff to be accurate.

In contrast, if you have very thin arms that measure 9 inches or less in circumference, you should use a special narrow cuff. These are also used for children, generally those below age twelve. In these cases, a regular cuff could give false readings much lower than the real blood pressure.

MEASURING YOUR OWN BLOOD PRESSURE AT HOME

Being able to monitor your blood pressure at home may be beneficial, but first ask your physician if he or she thinks it would be helpful or if it would make you too nervous about the usual hour-to-hour changes in blood pressure. You can purchase very adequate equipment for $30 to $90; more expensive models may be somewhat easier to use but are not necessarily more accurate. Do not make the mistake of buying a blood pressure cuff if you have no one to show you how to use it properly or repair it. Home blood pressure equipment and your measurement technique should be checked periodically in your doctor's office.

Make sure you have been sitting and are relatively relaxed for at least three to five minutes before measuring your blood pressure. This is to avoid measuring any brief increase in blood pressure that might be present if you just finished walking vigorously, smoking a cigarette, or drinking a cup of coffee; or if something had made you temporarily angry, nervous, or upset.

To measure your blood pressure, first use your finger to locate the beating of the pulse in the bend of your elbow. Straighten your arm and feel deep just inside the elbow tendon. When you feel the pulse, place the cuff on your arm so that the arrow on the cuff points toward the elbow artery (see Figure 2). Leave about one inch of space between the bottom part of the cuff and the bend of the elbow. Be sure none of your clothing is caught under the cuff since this could affect the reading.

Once the cuff is properly in place, take the rubber bulb of the blood pressure cuff in your hand and turn the screw valve to the right until it is closed. Then squeeze the bulb to pump up the cuff until you can no longer feel the pulse beat in your wrist, making note of the number on the gauge. This gives you a good idea of how high to pump up the cuff when you make your first measurement. Now turn the screw valve all the way to the left and let all the pressure out of the cuff until the gauge reads 0.

You are now ready to take your blood pressure. First, add thirty to the number that you saw on the gauge when the cuff blocked the pulse in your wrist. For example, if the pulse disappeared at 140 mm Hg, then you should pump the cuff up to 170 mm Hg.

Now place the stethoscope in your ears so that it fits comfortably. Put the listening end directly and firmly over the elbow artery but don't push too hard. Pump up the cuff to the level you determined, then slowly let the cuff pressure decrease by barely turning the screw valve to the left, so that the numbers on the gauge fall about 2 to 5 mm Hg per second. Write down the number when you hear the first of a continuing series of knocking sounds. This is the top number of the blood pressure, or the systolic blood pressure. Continue to slowly lessen the pressure of the cuff until the sound disappears completely. This is the bottom number of the blood pressure, or the diastolic blood pressure.

SPECIAL BLOOD PRESSURE
MEASUREMENT TECHNIQUES

Automatic Devices

Machines that automatically measure your blood pressure are available in many retail or drug stores. These devices are usually fairly accurate when tested in the laboratory. However, you may get a false reading if your arm does not fit well into the arm device, or you may have an elevated reading for a few minutes if you have been rushing around or carrying things. You should not change your blood pressure medicines based on these machine readings, but you should inform your physician if your reading is unexpectedly high, especially if you have new or worsening symptoms.

Ambulatory Blood Pressure Measurement

Equipment is now available that can automatically measure your blood pressure 4 to 150 times a day (including during your sleep) and record these values on machine-readable tapes. This information may be very useful for a few individuals who seem to have "yo-yo" blood pressure that suddenly goes way up and then way down for no obvious reason. It is also useful to detect those individuals whose blood pressure is high in the doctor's office but always normal at work or at home. This condition is referred to as "white coat" hypertension. The test is not done routinely, however, because it is not needed for most patients with high blood pressure and because it costs $125 to $250. All the reasons for using the device are still being researched.

Intraarterial Blood Pressure Measurement

The most accurate way to measure blood pressure is to put a needle in the artery and measure the pressure directly, rather than to estimate it from the cuff on the upper arm. This is not done routinely because it can be painful and because the cuff method is reasonably accurate. If you need to be hospitalized for dangerously high blood pressure, however, it may be necessary to measure and follow your exact blood pressure by this procedure, usually performed in an intensive care unit.

NEED FOR PERIODIC MEASUREMENT

Regular, accurate measurements are the only way to be certain your blood pressure is not high. Patients rarely have any symptoms to indicate they are hypertensive. Indeed, by the time certain symptoms do appear, they sometimes signal a medical emergency that requires immediate treatment. Regular blood pressure measurements and appropriate treatment can prevent such emergencies.

Healthy adults should have their blood pressure checked once a year. Persons at higher risk, such as those whose parents had hypertension or black adults over the age of forty, should have their blood pressure checked twice a year.

3

How Do You Feel with High Blood Pressure?

MILD TO MODERATE HIGH BLOOD PRESSURE

High blood pressure does not usually make you feel bad. As a matter of fact, most people who have high blood pressure feel fine, at least during the early stages of the disease. This is a mixed blessing. You can go about your day-to-day activities without any interference; however, the pressure is silently working against you by:

- increasing the work of the heart, making it pump harder and get larger and eventually weaker.
- decreasing the blood flow to your kidneys and heart, so that they do not receive proper nourishment.
- bursting or blocking a blood vessel in your brain, so that you have a stroke.

This is why high blood pressure is often called "the silent killer."

In a few cases, people report a feeling of giddiness or dizziness that may suggest high blood pressure, but the odds are high that you will feel fine. The only way you can determine whether you have high blood pressure is by having your pressure measured with a blood pressure cuff.

SEVERE HIGH BLOOD PRESSURE

If your blood pressure levels are extremely high, symptoms can occur, such as:

- nose bleed
- sudden temporary blindness
- shortness of breath
- chest pain
- dizziness
- severe pounding headache or pressure in the head

Most times, however, these problems are caused by something other than severe high blood pressure. For example, headaches can be caused by fever, migraine, anxiety, or infection. High blood pressure is not necessarily the culprit. Of course, if you suddenly feel worse or experience unusual symptoms, you should always check with your doctor. If you do have severe high blood pressure, it can be treated with strong medications, and the symptoms usually disappear.

Your doctor can determine if you need emergency

treatment by measuring your blood pressure to see how high it really is. Generally speaking, diastolic (lower number) blood pressures of 120 mm Hg or more need urgent referral and those of 130 mm Hg or more are considered particularly dangerous. Systolic (upper number) blood pressure levels of 210 mm Hg or more are also generally considered urgent and dangerous. Your own doctor may determine whether levels lower or higher than these are dangerous in your particular case, depending on many other clinical findings.

Your doctor can also look into your eyes with a special light (ophthalmoscope). If the blood pressure in your brain is extremely high, it will cause the nerves attached to your eyes to swell or the small blood vessels in the back of your eyes to burst. The doctor might also test a sample of your urine with a special paper strip to determine if your kidneys are losing protein; high levels of protein in the urine (proteinuria) indicate kidney damage. He or she may examine the urine under a microscope to see if there is any blood in it, which might indicate damage to some of the tiny blood vessels in the kidneys. All of these tests help the doctor determine whether your symptoms—headache, nose bleed, etc.—are because of severe high blood pressure.

SIDE EFFECTS FROM DRUGS

Occasionally, high blood pressure medicines can cause side effects. This was common with the earlier medicines, but occurs less frequently with the newer drugs. Chapter 11 discusses side effects in detail. If you are feeling bad, check with your doctor. But do not switch or stop medicines or lower the dose yourself—this could be dangerous.

FEELING GOOD

Most of the time, high blood pressure does not affect the way you feel. For this reason, you should never assume that you do not have high blood pressure because you have no symptoms. *You should never stop treatment just because you are feeling good or because your blood pressure is now "normal."* The most likely reason your blood pressure is "normal" is because your medicine is effective. If you feel fine after you have made certain recommended changes in your lifestyle—for example, lost weight, stopped smoking, reduced salt intake, began regular exercise—you should still check with your doctor regarding whether you can reduce the dose of your medicines or, in rare cases, stop medication altogether. But do not stop treatment by yourself. For the majority of people, once you have high blood pressure, you have it for life.

even higher when the high blood pressure is associated
between blood pressure, target-organ disease, and

4

What Are the Dangers of High Blood Pressure?

TARGET-ORGAN DAMAGE

High blood pressure is dangerous because if it is
not treated and controlled, it can damage important organs of the body: the heart, brain,
kidneys, and eyes. These are known as "target"
organs. When blood pressure remains abnormally
high for a long time, usually years, the increased
force against the walls of the arteries causes them to
become thicker and crooked, decreasing the flow of
blood to the heart, brain, kidneys, and eyes (Figure
3). As a result, these organs become damaged and
cannot function properly. If the damage is severe
enough, you can die.

In the United States and other westernized countries, cardiovascular (heart and blood vessel) disease
is the number one cause of death. Death rates are
higher when high blood pressure is also present and

even higher when the high blood pressure is associated with other risk factors such as cigarette smoking and high blood cholesterol.

The most common consequence of high blood pressure is heart attack. Figure 4 shows the relation between high blood pressure, heart disease, and stroke. It is quite certain that the unusually high death rate from strokes and heart attacks in the black community is very closely related to both the high rate of high blood pressure in this group and the relatively low rates of awareness, treatment, and control of this condition.

Heart

High blood pressure affects the heart in two ways: enlargement of the heart (cardiomegaly) and increased hardening, thickening, and blockage of the coronary arteries (arteriosclerosis). These changes can lead to chest pain (angina), heart attacks, heart failure, and irregular heartbeats (palpitations and flutters).

Heart Attack and Angina. Until high blood pressure damages the target organs, you usually will have no symptoms or physical complaints. If you develop coronary disease (i.e., hardening or blockage of the arteries that supply blood to the heart), however, you may feel severe chest pain as the result of a heart attack. This is when the blood flow to the heart is blocked and a part of the heart muscle dies from lack of nourishment. Or you may feel occasional chest pains, discomfort, pressure, or tightness usually brought on by exercise or emotional upset. These

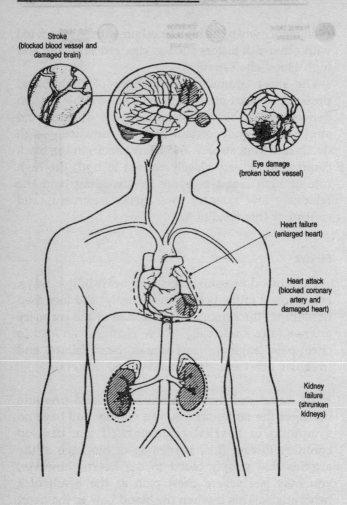

Stroke
(blocked blood vessel and
damaged brain)

Eye damage
(broken blood vessel)

Heart failure
(enlarged heart)

Heart attack
(blocked coronary
artery and
damaged heart)

Kidney
failure
(shrunken
kidneys)

Figure 3 COMPLICATIONS OF HIGH BLOOD PRESSURE

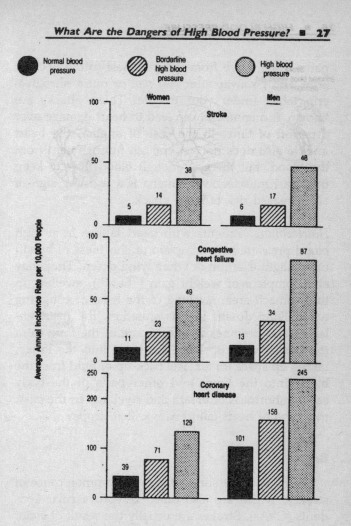

Figure 4 RELATION BETWEEN HIGH BLOOD PRESSURE, STROKE, CONGESTIVE HEART FAILURE AND CORONARY HEART DISEASE

pains often move from the midchest to the neck or arms and go away after you rest or put a nitroglycerin tablet under your tongue. These attacks are known as angina and can lead to heart damage over a period of time. In the case of angina, the heart muscle also does not get enough nourishment from the blood, but there is enough blood flow to keep the heart muscle alive. Angina is a warning sign of an increased risk of heart attack.

Heart Failure. Patients with heart failure from high blood pressure may complain of shortness of breath upon slight exertion or when lying down. They may also complain of weight gain ("fluid"), swelling in the stomach area, swelling of the legs, or coughing when lying down. In this situation, the heart enlarges and becomes weaker. Some of the fluid from the blood backs up from the heart into the lungs, taking up space for air. The back-up of fluid from the blood into the lungs and other parts of the body causes shortness of breath and swelling. In the past, this type of heart failure was called dropsy.

Brain

High blood pressure is the most common cause of strokes, which are also called cerebrovascular accidents (CVAs). Strokes are usually the result of a clot (thrombosis) in a blood vessel or a bursting of a blood vessel (hemorrhage) in the brain. This cuts off the supply of oxygen and nutrients, so that a portion of the brain gets sick and dies. Strokes can result in paralysis of one side of the body, difficulty in speaking or swallowing, blindness, mental confusion, sei-zures, and death. High blood pressure can cause a stroke in anyone, but the two highest risk groups are Japanese and blacks.

Fewer cases of stroke occur in young persons, and the stroke is not always related to high blood pressure. In some people, certain blood vessels in the brain have been weak since birth (congenital), and later in life these blood vessels balloon out to form blood-filled sacs (aneurysms) that can suddenly burst and cause a stroke.

Kidneys

Your kidneys filter waste substances out of the blood into the urine. If your kidneys do not function properly, these waste substances build up in the blood and, beyond a certain level, begin to poison your body.

As in the heart, the blood vessels in your kidneys can become hardened and thickened as a result of high blood pressure, and they cannot carry enough blood to nourish these organs and aid in eliminating waste. The result is kidney (renal) failure. When kidney failure causes generalized symptoms and ill-ness, it is known as uremia. Symptoms of early kidney failure are vague and not particularly related to the kidney itself. If the kidney were infected, you might feel pain in your side or lower back, have frequent urination, or feel a burning sensation when urinating. If the kidney failed, you might experience fatigue, weakness, nausea, vomiting, and/or mental depression.

If you were to develop severe kidney failure, you would need to undergo dialysis and be "on a machine" several times a week to remove body waste and stay alive. Death will often occur if dialysis cannot be done or if it fails because of infection or other complications. Sometimes dialysis may be temporary and in suitable patients with proper donor kidneys, can be replaced by transplantation of one kidney.

Eyes

Long-standing high blood pressure can cause serious eye problems, such as bleeding (retinal hemorrhage) or clots in the small eye vessels or tearing away of the lining of the inner eye (detached retinas). Again, these problems result from blood vessel damage caused by high blood pressure. These eye complications can cause no symptoms or they can cause blindness, depending on the exact location of the problem in the eye. When diabetes, commonly found in combination with high blood pressure, has caused eye problems, the high blood pressure can make the eye complications worse.

YOUR RISKS ARE UNNECESSARY

What we have said so far sounds very alarming, but there is good news. While high blood pressure can damage the heart, brain, kidneys, and eyes (target organs), controlling your blood pressure so that it does not remain abnormally high for long periods of time can help prevent the damage. Indeed, the treatment of high blood pressure has resulted in dramatic decreases in the rates of sickness and death. Although this is true for all cardiovascular diseases complicated by high blood pressure, the improvement has been most dramatic in the frequency of strokes. In the United States, the stroke rate has been declining for the past thirty to thirty-five years, especially since the availability of more public-education programs and the discovery of some better-tolerated and more effective drugs for high blood pressure.

5

Who Treats High Blood Pressure?

GENERAL PHYSICIANS OR SPECIALISTS?

Doctors in many different areas of medicine are trained to treat high blood pressure. General practitioners (GPs), family practitioners, internists, pediatricians, cardiologists (heart experts), and nephrologists (kidney experts) are only some examples.

In unusual cases in which there are special causes for the high blood pressure or if the usual medicines are not working, a second opinion from a specialist may be appropriate. Your particular case would determine the type of specialist. If the kidneys were the main organ affected, then your doctor would probably recommend a nephrologist; if the heart were affected, a cardiologist. A few advanced medical research and training programs enable doctors to spend many years specializing in high blood pressure, but there is not a separate specialty for "hypertensionologists."

High blood pressure is not a rare disease as are certain illnesses for which sophisticated medical centers provide highly specialized care. It is a common problem with standard approaches to treatment that are accepted by most medical groups.

In general, the diagnosis and treatment of high blood pressure is not very complicated. Most doctors involved in primary care of patients are well qualified to treat your condition. In most cases, you are likely to have no problems and live a long and healthy life. There is no reason to lose a lot of sleep, worry endlessly, or shop around for a different opinion if you are feeling well and your blood pressure is controlled. If your doctor tells you that you have high blood pressure, then relax and take it easy—but take it seriously. If you visit your doctor as he or she instructs, take your medicines as directed, and follow instructions for diet, smoking, etc., you should do fine. But you will have to follow instructions carefully, take responsibility for doing all you can, and be an active participant in your own health care.

Often doctors work with nurse practitioners or physician assistants to help manage high blood pressure patients. These therapists have received extensive health education and training, and often have more time to spend with you than your doctor does. They can go into greater detail answering your questions about tests and medications and various lifestyle changes, including diet and exercise. This team effort has proven to be successful.

PUBLIC HEALTH PROGRAMS

High blood pressure is a major public health problem. If high blood pressure were detected and controlled in everyone, we could save tens of thousands of lives and save billions of dollars each year in medical costs and lost workdays. For this reason, governments and private foundations have funded major community, national, and international programs for high blood pressure screening and education. These programs identify people who don't know they have high blood pressure, educate them about the disease, and refer them for care.

Certain programs provide ongoing follow-up evaluations or treatment for those who cannot afford high blood pressure care. You probably can find free blood-pressure check sites and educational programs at churches, barbershops, drugstores, fire stations, your place of work, neighborhood community centers, public health departments, dentists' offices, podiatry offices, and many other locations in your community. The local American Heart Association, National Kidney Foundation, or County Medical Society may also be able to assist you in locating such a blood pressure program. If your blood pressure is elevated or above "normal" at a blood pressure check location, you should see your doctor to confirm the diagnosis of high blood pressure and the need for treatment. Very high levels require immediate attention.

There are also regional, national, and international conferences on high blood pressure. Some are for the public at large. You might be able to find out about such conferences by contacting your local hospital or medical school.

There are also centers funded by national governments or the World Health Organization. Many of these, such as the National High Blood Pressure Education Program in Bethesda, Maryland, provide free literature and library resources for the general public (see Appendix III).

6

What Are the Usual Examinations and Tests for High Blood Pressure?

THE HISTORY

Chief Complaint

Everyone who goes to a physician is used to a certain routine, beginning with the question, "What is your problem?" or "Why did you come in to see me?" Physicians call your answer to this question the "chief complaint." It is the first part of the patient history that the physician records on your chart before starting the examination.

In the case of high blood pressure, you are not likely to have a chief symptom or complaint unless your blood pressure is extremely high or is causing your heart, kidneys, or brain to function abnormally. Most patients who develop high blood pressure do not go to see their physician because they are feeling bad. Instead, they discover their elevated blood pressure during a regular checkup or routine examination for insurance or a job, or at a screening program at a blood donation station, health fair, dentist's office, church, barbershop, drugstore, or other location offering community health programs. Once the measurements show their blood pressure is up, then they go to see the physician.

Blood Pressure History

Your doctor will ask questions to determine if, in the past, you had elevated blood pressure that later returned to normal, as can happen during pregnancy, or you were ever diagnosed as having high blood pressure. The physician may also be interested in any symptoms such as sweating spells, heart flutters, and sudden elevation of blood pressure that might suggest that the hypertension is caused by a rare condition, such as a tumor of the adrenal gland (pheochromocytoma), which might be corrected by surgery.

Family and Personal History

Your doctor will also be interested in whether your parents or other relatives have had high blood pressure or any of its complications: stroke, heart attack, etc. He will ask about risk factors such as cigarette smoking, high blood cholesterol, eating habits, diabetes, amount of exercise, stress, or nervous conditions and other factors that, combined with high blood pressure, can increase your chance of heart attack.

Medications and Other Substances

You will also be asked what medicines you are taking, including over-the-counter medicines and those prescribed by physicians. Your answers are important because certain drugs taken for colds, allergies, or nasal stuffiness contain chemicals that can make high blood pressure worse; for example, chemicals such as pseudoephedrine, phenylpropanolamine, or phenylephrine are commonly found in many such remedies. Some prescription drugs can also sometimes make it more difficult to control your high blood pressure if you are taking blood pressure drugs; for example, birth control pills and anti-arthritis drugs can raise blood pressure (see Chapter 10). Certain over-the-counter medicines contain high quantities of salt (sodium), which can increase your blood pressure. In addition, excessive amounts of certain other substances such as chewing tobacco and licorice can also elevate your blood pressure. Obviously, the physician will want to explore all of these possibilities.

THE PHYSICAL EXAMINATION

Next, the physician will do a physical examination, which has four main purposes:

- to determine by several measurements what the blood pressure is,
- to determine how much, if any, damage has been done to the heart, eyes, brain, kidneys, blood vessels, etc. (target organs),

- to look for any signs of the type of high blood pressure that can be corrected by surgery (secondary hypertension), and
- to determine if there are any clinical reasons to choose one blood pressure medicine over another.

Blood Pressure

On the first visit, your doctor usually will want to check the pressure in both arms, as well as in the lying or sitting, and standing positions. Blood pressure is generally the same in both arms or a little higher in the right arm, but a big difference could indicate a narrowing of the main blood vessel coming off the heart, known as coarctation of the aorta, a rare cause of high blood pressure. Occasionally, blood pressure should be measured in the legs if this condition (coarctation) is suspected. If you stand up, it is normal for the systolic blood pressure (top number) to drop a little and the diastolic blood pressure (bottom number) to increase a little. Certain drugs, however, can alter the standing blood pressure. For example, drugs that affect the nervous system sometimes cause blood pressure to drop substantially when the patient stands up, but reduce blood pressure less when the patient is sitting or lying down. The pulse rate should also be measured carefully during the examination because it, too, can be changed by various blood pressure drugs.

Sometimes the physician will measure your blood pressure after exercise, and before and after you start taking drugs to treat your hypertension. If you are very active, he or she may want to bring your blood pressure down to a lower level at rest in order to avoid dangerous increases during exercise.

Eyes

One of the most important parts of the physical examination of a hypertensive patient is the eye examination. When the physician looks through your pupil with a device called an ophthalmoscope, he or she sees small blood vessels (arterioles) that tend to vary in size and crookedness according to the severity of your high blood pressure and the length of time you have had it. Very narrowed, crooked vessels can be found in cases of long-standing high blood pressure. If the blood pressure problem is very severe, bleeding points (hemorrhages) and fluid collections (exudates) appear on the back of the eye (eye ground) and often indicate the need for urgent treatment. In rare cases, extremely severe high blood pressure can produce swelling of the nerve to the eye (papilledema), which can cause blindness. With successful treatment, however, vision usually returns to normal.

Heart

The heart examination is always an important part of the physical examination of a hypertensive patient. The physician looks for any enlargement of the heart, unusual heart sounds (gallops), murmurs, or irregular heartbeats (palpitations) to determine if long-standing or severely elevated blood pressure has caused any damage to this vital organ. Sometimes, if the blood pressure problem has gone untreated for a long time, the heart will enlarge and grow weaker. Eventually the heart becomes too weak to pump blood effectively through the body, and heart failure occurs, causing shortness of breath and swelling of the legs. Excess fluid (edema) collects in your lungs, abdomen, and legs.

If the blood vessels to the heart become hardened and blocked (coronary disease), you could suffer a heart attack. Whether or not you have had a heart attack does not necessarily show up on the physical examination, so your doctor may have to perform special tests such as an electrocardiogram (EKG) to help make this diagnosis.

Abdomen

The physician examines your abdomen carefully by feeling for masses that could indicate you have an enlarged kidney, a tumor of the adrenal gland, or a ballooning (aneurysm) of the main artery (aorta) leading from the heart. Any of these findings could be a result of high blood pressure (secondary hypertension). The physician also listens with the stethoscope for swishing noises (bruits) in the stomach area. These can be the first indication of a partially blocked artery to the kidney, which can cause high blood pressure.

Legs and Feet

To examine the blood vessels in the leg, the physician places his or her fingers over the arteries in your legs and feet. This allows the doctor to determine if blood flow through these vessels has been decreased by hardening of the arteries (arteriosclerosis), which occurs more frequently in people with high blood pressure.

Nervous System

An examination of your nervous system includes checking your reflexes, balance, and strength. It determines if you show any evidence of impaired movement, feeling, speaking, thinking, or other functions of your body that are controlled by the brain. These findings could indicate that you have had a stroke in the past. Strokes occur more frequently in persons with untreated high blood pressure. Small strokes (mini-strokes) can occur with temporary loss of some of the functions just mentioned. These are very important and should be reported immediately to your doctor because early diagnosis and treatment can prevent a more serious massive stroke with permanent disability or death.

LABORATORY STUDIES

Whereas the history given by the patient and the examination done by the physician contribute the most to medical diagnosis, laboratory studies serve to confirm certain suspicions. They occasionally add information not obtained by the history and physical examination.

Urinalysis

Because high blood pressure is often related to the kidneys, a urine examination is usually done when you are first evaluated. If protein or red blood cells are present in the urine, this often indicates that the kidneys have been damaged, either by primary disease or by long-standing untreated high blood pressure. High blood pressure can also cause the kidneys to produce a "weak" (dilute) urine. Occasionally, other findings from the urinalysis will point to a cause for high blood pressure that might be cured by surgery.

Blood Chemistries

Laboratory tests measure the levels of certain substances in your blood, determine if any organs are functioning abnormally, and provide a basis from which to monitor the effects of drugs. Blood studies for hypertension include tests for sodium, potassium, chloride, and CO_2 (electrolytes) and tests for blood urea nitrogen (BUN) and creatinine. If the blood potassium is found to be low before drugs are given, this can indicate a rare tumor of the adrenal gland (aldosteronoma) that can cause high blood pressure. Much more often, low potassium is caused by diuretic drugs used as part of your treatment. An elevation in two tests, the BUN and creatinine, often indicates damage to your kidneys from high blood pressure. Occasionally, these values can also be elevated if a kidney problem is causing your high blood pressure or if you have become dehydrated.

Additional blood studies—including tests for blood sugar (glucose), cholesterol, and uric acid—can identify other risks for developing heart problems (cardiovascular risk factors). Since the levels of these chemicals in the blood can be changed by some of the drugs used to treat high blood pressure, their measurement is important before you begin treatment. The tests are repeated periodically while you continue to take medications.

Blood Count

A blood count, often known as a CBC (complete blood count), will determine if the patient has an abnormal red or white blood-cell count. This is a generally accepted, good health test to make sure that you don't have other conditions such as anemia, a low red blood-cell count. In addition, it is an important baseline measurement to monitor the effects of certain high blood pressure medications (see Chapter 11).

Electrocardiogram and Chest X-ray

The electrocardiogram (EKG) and chest X-ray help determine more precisely the degree of heart damage that may have resulted from your high blood pressure. The physician can also use the EKG to observe the influence of drug therapy on the heart. The EKG can detect marked enlargement of the heart and any abnormal function of certain parts of the heart (e.g., the atrium) that resulted from longstanding high blood pressure. Abnormal or irregular beating of the heart, sometimes found with high blood pressure, can also be detected and defined better by the EKG than by the physical examination alone.

Probably the most important value of the EKG is for the diagnosis of coronary artery disease (heart attack and angina), which is the most common complication of high blood pressure and the number one cause of death in the Western world. For this reason, the EKG has special value in the evaluation and management of patients with high blood pressure. The EKG does not always detect evidence of a previous heart attack, however, and it is possible to have dangerous heart disease with a normal EKG.

The chest X-ray is especially useful in assessing heart enlargement and diagnosing heart failure. When heart failure resulting from high blood pressure is treated, the chest X-ray is one of the best ways to follow its improvement. The chest X-ray also shows other structures in the chest, such as the aorta and other arteries, the lungs, and the air passages of the lungs that relate to high blood pressure.

SUMMARY

We have presented a description of how we and other physicians examine a patient with high blood pressure, how we arrive at and confirm the diagnosis, how we proceed to assess the extent of damage to various organs of the body, and finally, how the physical examination and laboratory studies help us monitor good and bad effects from hypertension treatment. As always, if you have any questions about your own examination and tests, ask your doctor.

7

Are There Special Tests for People with High Blood Pressure?

The preceding chapter described the tests that are done often on patients with high blood pressure; this chapter describes special tests used less frequently. These tests are performed only if you are one of the unusual cases with certain symptoms or findings on your routine evaluation indicating a possible secondary cause for high blood pressure.

KIDNEY TESTS

Intravenous Pyelogram (IVP)

The IVP is an X-ray test that helps your physician determine whether a kidney problem may be causing your elevated blood pressure. Dye injected through a needle into the vein of your arm travels to your kidneys and shows up on a series of X-ray pictures taken over a period of thirty minutes or so. You may experience a brief hot or flushed feeling from the dye, and there is a slight chance you could get a skin rash if you are allergic to the dye. The test can help identify whether you are one of the 5 to 10 percent of people whose hypertension is caused by a kidney problem, although it is only about 70 percent accurate. For example, one kidney might be smaller as the result of past infections or a blocked blood flow. Two very large kidneys usually means polycystic kidney disease, a particular type of problem inherited in your family.

Arteriogram (Angiogram)

An arteriogram involves kidney X-rays similar to the IVP except that the dye is injected into one of the arteries in your groin. The test is more uncomfortable than the IVP but more accurate because it directly shows whether or not there is narrowing of the blood vessels (arteries) that lead to your kidney. If one of your kidney blood vessels is too narrow, it can cause high blood pressure, which can be cured by widening the artery. Methods used to widen the artery include balloon angioplasty or surgery. In angioplasty, a small balloon is blown up within the narrow interior of the artery. If necessary, abdominal surgery can improve the blood supply to the artery by bypassing the narrowed vessel with a piece of vein from your leg (saphenous vein bypass) or with a piece of artificial tubing (Dacron patch graft) that brings blood directly to the kidney from the main blood vessel of the body, the aorta.

Digital Subtraction Angiography (DSA)

A digital subtraction angiogram outlines the kidney blood vessels by either injecting dye through a vein (venous DSA) or an artery (arterial DSA). The method uses special computerized X-ray techniques (digital subtraction). Less dye is needed than with an arteriogram, but the DSA is slightly less accurate.

HEART TESTS

Echocardiogram (ECHO)

An echocardiogram is a painless test in which sound waves are bounced off the heart and shown on a TV screen. The test is a sensitive indicator of the thickness of the walls of the heart. In particular, it shows whether high blood pressure has caused the left side of the heart to thicken excessively, a condition known as left ventricular hypertrophy, or LVH. The normal thickness of the relaxed left side of the heart is less than one-half inch. In LVH, it can thicken to more than an inch. The ECHO also measures how wide the chambers of the heart are, how well the heart contracts, and whether the heart valves are working normally without being stiff or leaky.

Holter Monitor

The Holter monitor is a twenty-four-hour-long electrocardiogram (EKG) to detect whether you have periods of strain on your heart or irregular heartbeats (arrhythmias) during your usual activities or sleep. It may reveal abnormalities that could not be found during the approximately two-minute test period of the resting EKG. In the Holter test, adhesive patches are placed on your chest and connected by wires to a battery-operated tape recorder that you wear around your neck.

Treadmill Exercise

The treadmill test may be done if you have chest discomfort that could be caused by poor circulation to the heart. This type of chest pain is called angina or angina pectoris. The test is usually done in a laboratory using a machine that can go slow or fast and that can tilt at different angles. Walking on such a treadmill is similar to trying to go up a down escalator. The exercise causes a normal increase in your heartbeat, and a constantly running EKG detects if the blood supply to your heart remains adequate during the extra stress of exercise. Often the treadmill test is coupled with an isotopic (thallium) scan to visualize the uptake of blood by different regions of the heart. If the results of your treadmill exercise test are normal, it is unlikely that your chest pain is caused by coronary artery disease, but it does not absolutely exclude this possibility. Conversely, if telltale signs of poor heart circulation (ischemia) appear on the EKG, it suggests that your chest pain _might_ be caused by coronary artery disease. In this case, you may need additional special tests.

OTHER SPECIAL TESTS

Twenty-Four-Hour Urine Collections

A twenty-four-hour urine collection is sometimes requested for patients with high blood pressure. You are asked to empty your bladder, discard the urine, note the time, then place all subsequent urine into a jug until that exact time the next day. Chemical analysis of the urine usually gives a fairly precise estimate of whether your kidneys are working normally or whether they are losing too much protein, a condition called proteinuria. It can also provide information on the usual amounts of minerals that you eat, such as sodium, potassium, and calcium. Sometimes it is used to measure specific hormones that are rare causes of high blood pressure. These special urinary hormones include catecholamines, metanephrine, and vanillylmandelic acid (VMA). An elevation of these substances could indicate the presence of a usually noncancerous tumor that produces adrenaline-like substances that raise blood pressure in conjunction with profuse sweating, pounding headaches, and a fast heartbeat.

Special Blood Tests
(Thyroid Hormone, Renin, Catecholamines, Aldosterone)

Special blood tests are sometimes done to measure certain hormones or substances that could be contributing to your high blood pressure. For example, an overactive thyroid gland with high blood levels of thyroid hormone can cause high blood pressure.

Renin is another blood substance that is associated with high blood pressure. The kidneys produce renin whenever they do not get an adequate supply of blood. The renin then causes blood vessels to clamp down and blood pressure to rise. Therefore, a high level of renin in the blood could indicate that your high blood pressure is caused by blocked or reduced blood flow to your kidney, and that you may need specific X-rays of these kidney arteries (a renal arteriogram or DSA).

About one out of every five to ten patients with high blood pressure has unexplained high levels of renin. In this special situation, the blood pressure responds unusually well to such drugs as Accupril, Altace, Capoten, Lotensin, Monopril, Prinivil, Vasotec, or Zestril. Black patients with high blood pressure, older patients, and diabetics often have low blood levels of renin. Blood pressure in this situation often responds well to such drugs as Adalat, Calan, Cardene, Cardizem, Dyazide, DynaCirc, Hydrochlorothiazide (HCTZ), Hygroton, Isoptin, Lasix, Lozol, Maxzide, Norvasc, Plendil, Procardia, and Verelan.

About one in every one thousand hypertensive patients has a rare condition called pheochromocytoma.

This occurs when the tiny adrenal gland just above the kidney produces too many adrenaline-like hormones called catecholamines. At least three of these hormones (norepinephrine, epinephrine, and dopamine) can be measured in the blood, and extremely high levels indicate a need to further examine this gland, usually by obtaining a computerized axial tomography (CAT) scan of the abdomen.

Tumors of the adrenal gland can also produce too much of the hormone aldosterone. Excess amounts of aldosterone can cause elevated blood pressure and loss of potassium into the urine, resulting in low levels of potassium in the blood (hypokalemia) that can lead to profound muscle weakness and serious rhythm problems of the heart.

8

Are There Causes for High Blood Pressure That Can Be Cured?

High blood pressure is not like pneumonia, a condition that goes away after you receive a shot and take pills for a couple of weeks. High blood pressure is a chronic disease and, in most cases, you will need to take medication for life. Patients often mistakenly assume that their blood pressure is cured after they go to the doctor and begin taking medications that bring the pressure down to normal. Unfortunately, the dosages of the medicines available today last for 8 to 12 hours, or a few days at most. In most cases, if you stop your medication, your blood pressure will bounce back up as high as or even higher than it was originally. Therefore, one of the most important things to learn is that, for most people, high blood pressure is a problem you will have for life, yet it should not bother you as long as you take your medicine.

Only a few people who have high blood pressure

do not have to take medications for the rest of their lives. Some have it only because they are overweight. A small number of them are willing and able to lose the excess weight. And an even smaller number keep the weight off. So it is dangerous to say, "There's no need for me to take drugs. I'll just lose weight and my blood pressure will come down." If you do not lose the weight, your blood pressure will remain elevated, and you will continue to be at risk of having a stroke or developing heart disease and kidney disease. If you actually were to lose weight and keep it off, you would still need to have your blood pressure checked every few months to make certain that, in fact, your blood pressure had returned to normal levels and was staying there.

Chapter 9 describes other changes in the way you live that may help control your blood pressure or problems associated with high blood pressure. These lifestyle changes relate to salt, alcohol, potassium, calcium, cholesterol and fat, smoking, exercise, and stress. These approaches are only used as sole therapy for patients with mildly elevated blood pressure, but they are quite useful in addition to drug therapy for the majority of patients with high blood pressure.

SECONDARY HYPERTENSION

Approximately 5 to 10 percent of people with high blood pressure have the condition because of specific abnormalities, such as high levels of certain substances in the blood, tumors (usually noncancerous), irregularities in the blood vessels, or kidney disease. Once the underlying condition is corrected, blood pressure returns to normal.

Licorice and Chewing Tobacco

Licorice, either in candy or chewing tobacco, can cause your body to retain salt and raise your blood pressure. This does not happen to every person who chews tobacco or eats licorice, but it can occur if you use large amounts and are predisposed to developing high blood pressure.

Certain Medicines

Some drugs that your doctor may prescribe for you, such as prednisone, cyclosporine, estrogen-containing birth control pills, or nasal decongestants for colds, occasionally can raise your blood pressure.

Hormones

High blood pressure can also be caused by excessively high levels of hormones produced by various sources within your body. For example, a very rare, usually noncancerous tumor called pheo (short for pheochromocytoma) may grow just above your kidney and produce an adrenaline-like substance that can suddenly raise your blood pressure, make your heart beat rapidly (palpitations), and give you headaches. If your doctor feels that you might have this unusual problem, he or she will order certain tests: blood tests (catecholamines), urine tests (VMA or metanephrine), X-rays (dye studies called angiograms), and/or CAT scans (more sophisticated X-rays). If you are found to have one of these unusual tumors, a surgeon can usually operate and remove it, and your blood pressure probably will return to normal.

A tumor or enlargement of the pituitary gland in the brain or the adrenal gland above your kidneys could also be the culprit. Different blood and urine tests as well as X-rays and scans evaluate this possibility. You might have a low blood level of potassium or renin (see Chapter 7) or a high level of cortisol (Cushing's syndrome), a substance made by the adrenal gland. If a small extra part of the adrenal gland has become overdeveloped (adenoma), it can often be removed surgically. If both adrenal glands are enlarged, medications may be appropriate. Special "water pills" that cause the kidneys to retain potassium may also be useful.

Pregnancy

Approximately one out of every twenty women can develop high blood pressure during the last three months of pregnancy. The high blood pressure usually causes symptoms such as sudden weight gain, swelling of the feet and legs, headache, spots in front of the eyes, and stomach pains. Temporary blindness and kidney failure occur rarely.

This condition has a variety of names: toxemia, preeclampsia, and pregnancy-induced hypertension. If convulsions (i.e., seizures or epilepsy) occur, it is called eclampsia. The cause is unknown but it is more likely to occur in women:

- who are pregnant for the first time
- who have diabetes
- who are carrying twins
- whose mother or sister had the same condition
- who have not had regular medical checkups during their pregnancy

Cigarette smoking during pregnancy does not cause toxemia, but it does make it more likely that the baby will have a lower-than-expected birth weight, or that the baby may be premature and weigh less than 5½ pounds.

If the elevation of blood pressure is mild, it can usually be treated with hospitalization and bed rest. Lying down on the left side is especially useful to help keep the blood pressure controlled, perhaps because it relieves some of the pressure that the womb puts on blood vessels. More severe cases may require medications such as Aldomet, Apresoline, or shots of magnesium sulfate. In rare cases, the blood pressure is so high and hard to treat that the pregnancy has to be terminated in order to save the mother.

The mother's elevated blood pressure will almost always return to normal within a few days after delivery of the baby. However, a few women with repeated bouts of toxemia will get chronic hypertension that requires lifelong therapy.

Toxemia is a serious condition, but death is rare unless convulsions occur. However, the risk of death is more than doubled for the baby when the mother has toxemia, and many of the babies born alive are much smaller than expected.

Narrowing of the Main Artery

If the main blood vessel (aorta) coming from your heart is very narrow at a specific point, it can increase the blood pressure in your arms and lower the blood pressure in your legs. This happens because the aorta narrows after it supplies blood to the arms but before it supplies blood to the legs (see Figure 5).

A simple way to understand this is to think of your garden hose with water coming out the nozzle. If you stepped on the hose, the pressure would build up between the spigot and your foot, as it does in the arm blood vessels, but the pressure would decrease between your foot and the nozzle, as in the blood vessels in the leg. The doctor may check this problem by taking your leg blood pressure and your arm blood pressure. He or she may order X-ray dye studies of the aorta. This condition (coarctation of the aorta) is usually found in very young children and can be treated with surgery.

Narrowing of Kidney Arteries

As discussed in Chapter 7, blood tests for renin, a substance produced in the kidneys, and X-rays (IVP and arteriogram) can be helpful in diagnosing the narrowing of one or more of your kidney arteries that causes high blood pressure (renovascular hypertension). The doctor may listen with the stethoscope and hear a swishing sound (bruit) in the stomach area, where the blood rushes through the narrowed spot. Procedures to cure this narrowing include

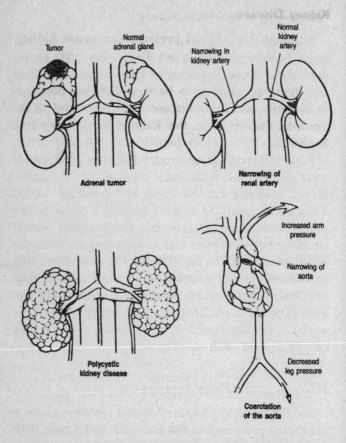

Figure 5 CAUSES OF HIGH BLOOD PRESSURE THAT CAN BE CURED

angioplasty—placing a small tube with a small balloon into the vessel, and then inflating the balloon to open the narrowed portion—or surgically implanting a new blood vessel that detours the blood around the narrowed spot in the renal artery.

Kidney Disease

Although high blood pressure can cause kidney disease, kidney disease can also cause high blood pressure. As a matter of fact, as many as 5 percent of all hypertensive patients have high blood pressure as a result of kidney disease. Infections and other diseases that damage the kidneys (e.g., diabetes, nephritis, or lupus erythematosus) can also cause hypertension.

Diet Pills

An overdose of diet pills that contain stimulants known as amphetamines can cause severe elevation of blood pressure and even stroke. Patients with high blood pressure should not take any type of diet pill that has not been prescribed or approved by their physician.

Street Drugs

Use of cocaine or street drugs called speed can also cause extreme elevations of blood pressure, stroke, and heart attack. Cocaine abuse is often associated with high blood pressure, chest pain, and seizures ("fits").

SUMMARY

The doctor determines whether to evaluate you for all or some of these possible causes of high blood pressure with the understanding that they are not common and that many of the tests are expensive and can cause complications. The choice should be a decision made by you and your doctor together. You should feel comfortable talking with your doctor and asking any questions you may have. How many tests should be performed to look for specific causes of your high blood pressure? When should you change medicines because of a side effect? Talking about these issues avoids problems, improves your relationship with the doctor, and leads to more effective treatment.

9

Can Changes in the Way You Live Help Control Your Blood Pressure?

Can changes in the way you live help control your blood pressure? In many cases, yes. Even though we do not know what causes "essential" high blood pressure, we have proof that there are many factors associated with its development, such as age, race, and family history. Many of these cannot be controlled or prevented; however, weight, diet, and lifestyle can be controlled to a great extent, and their control may help prevent or reduce your high blood pressure.

This chapter describes what you can do for yourself to help control your blood pressure. This is not to suggest that you should treat yourself without a doctor. Once high blood pressure is suspected or diagnosed, you should continue to see your physician. He or she will do an evaluation and then prescribe treatment that will control the blood pressure and help prevent serious complications, such as stroke, heart attack, or kidney disease.

Most physicians now accept that there should be both drug treatment and nondrug treatment for high blood pressure. The great majority of hypertensive patients will require ongoing medication to control their blood pressure; however, nondrug treatment is sometimes effective when used alone in patients with mild hypertension. In addition, nondrug treatment can be combined with drug therapy to reduce the number and amounts of drugs needed to achieve control.

Although treatment is prescribed by the physician, it is your responsibility to follow directions. Ultimately, you play a very important role in controlling your high blood pressure. No amount of expertise on the part of your physician and no drug, however "miraculous," can do a thing if you do not learn about your condition, take your medicines, and make the necessary changes in how you live. Once you start, you will discover that you get results, that your blood pressure goes down, and that you can help control your condition. And once you see and feel those results, you will want to do even more to improve your health. This cooperation on your part is known as compliance. Lack of compliance represents a major problem in achieving blood pressure control. To benefit from treatment and protect your health, you should constantly commit yourself to taking your medications as prescribed, keeping your doctor appointments faithfully, and following the nondrug part of the treatment.

The two most important approaches to lower blood pressure are to lose weight and restrict your intake of salt.

WEIGHT

The association between high blood pressure and excess body weight has been noted for many years. You are considered overweight if you weigh more than 115 percent of your desirable body weight (see Table 2). For example, if you are a woman 5 feet, 4 inches tall and have a small body frame, your desirable body weight is approximately 120 pounds (halfway between 114 and 127), and overweight would be 120 x 1.15 or 138 pounds. If your ideal body weight is 190 pounds, overweight would be 190 x 1.15 or 219 pounds.

More cases of high blood pressure are found among obese or overweight people than among normal weight or underweight people. This does not mean that all overweight people have high blood pressure, nor does it mean that people who are not overweight avoid this condition. In most cases, however, people who either have high blood pressure or are at special risk of developing it are strongly advised to try to achieve and maintain ideal body weight. Even a small weight reduction can be beneficial if you are overweight. As little as ten pounds of weight loss can have a definite beneficial effect on blood pressure.

Anyone who has high blood pressure or would like to try to prevent it should eat properly and exercise regularly. Even twenty minutes of walking briskly, three times a week, could noticeably benefit your blood pressure. It is beyond the scope of this book to cover the details of special weight-reduction diets or other methods of weight loss, but we have

TABLE 2. Desirable Weights for Men and Women* [Weights at age 25-29 based on lowest mortality. Weight in pounds according to frame (in indoor clothing weighing 5 pounds for men and 3 pounds for women; shoes with 1-inch heels)]

MEN

Height Feet	Inches	Small Frame	Medium Frame	Large Frame
5	2	128-134	131-141	138-150
5	3	130-136	133-143	140-153
5	4	132-138	135-145	142-156
5	5	134-140	137-148	144-160
5	6	136-142	139-151	146-164
5	7	138-145	142-154	149-168
5	8	140-148	145-157	152-172
5	9	142-151	148-160	155-176
5	10	144-154	151-163	158-180
5	11	146-157	154-166	161-184
6	0	149-160	157-170	164-188
6	1	152-164	160-174	168-192
6	2	155-168	164-178	172-197
6	3	158-172	167-182	176-202
6	4	162-176	171-187	181-207

WOMEN

Height		Small	Medium	Large
Feet	Inches	Frame	Frame	Frame
4	10	102-111	109-121	118-131
4	11	103-113	111-123	120-134
5	0	104-115	113-128	122-137
5	1	106-118	115-129	125-140
5	2	108-121	118-132	128-143
5	3	111-124	121-135	131-147
5	4	114-127	124-138	134-151
5	5	117-130	127-141	137-155
5	6	120-133	130-144	140-159
5	7	123-136	133-147	143-163
5	8	126-139	136-150	146-167
5	9	129-142	139-153	149-170
5	10	132-145	142-156	152-173
5	11	135-148	145-159	155-176
6	0	138-151	148-162	158-179

*Metropolitan Life Insurance Company Health and Safety Education Division, 1983.

included a sample 1800-calorie diet from the American Heart Association to give you an idea of what kind of diet you might need to follow (Table 3). An 1800-calorie diet may only allow you to maintain your current weight. Lower amounts (i.e., 800 to 1200 calories) might be necessary for effective weight reduction. In addition, following some of the very simple dietary guidelines listed below will help you to lose weight.

Your doctor may recommend that you see a dietitian or nutritionist who can work with you to develop a diet suited to your individual needs that will be enjoyable as well as nutritious. Health departments and Health Maintenance Organizations (HMOs) also have dietitians and information available to help you develop a healthy diet plan.

Many books on this subject as well as different types of self-help groups are also available to you. Your doctor should be the one to refer you and approve the program you follow.

As you think about developing your own weight-loss plan and reducing your blood pressure levels, keep these simple principles in mind:

- Eat less red meat. When you do eat red meat, choose the leaner cuts, trim off the fat, and broil or bake instead of frying the meat.
- Eat more fish and chicken. Broil or bake instead of frying, and consider taking the skin off.
- Avoid sugar and sweets. These include honey, jellies, jams, syrups, molasses, cakes, and candies. Cut down on the number of desserts you

TABLE 3. Sample Two-Day Menus for an
1800-Calorie Diet

DAY 1	DAY 2
Breakfast	**Breakfast**
2 medium prunes with 2 tablespoons juice ¾ cup puffed wheat 1 cup milk 1 slice toast; 1 small pat butter Coffee or tea, if desired	½ cup grapefruit juice 1 medium egg, scrambled ½ cup applesauce 2 slices toast; 1 small pat butter Coffee or tea, if desired
Mid-morning snack	**Mid-morning snack**
½ cup milk	½ cup milk 5 crackers (two-inch square)
Lunch	**Lunch**
2 ounces broiled liver Baked acorn squash with 1 small pat butter Cabbage slaw with caraway seeds, green pepper, and vinegar 2 medium muffins; 1 small pat butter Apricot bread pudding made with 1 slice bread, 1 small pat butter, 4 dried apricot halves, and ¼ cup milk Coffee or tea, if desired	2 ounces sliced roast chicken ⅓ cup bread dressing 1 tablespoon cranberry sauce ½ cup cauliflower Lettuce salad 1 medium roll; 1 small pat butter Coffee or tea, if desired
Mid-afternoon snack	**Mid-afternoon snack**
1 small orange	1 small pear Coffee or tea, if desired

DAY 1	DAY 2
Dinner	**Dinner**
Baked casserole of beef with whipped potato topping made with 3 ounces cooked beef, ½ cup broth from beef, and ½ cup potato	Homemade bean soup made with ½ cup dried beans
	2 ounces broiled halibut with lemon
Green beans	½ cup green peas
Tomato and cucumber salad on lettuce with 1 tablespoon French dressing	1 small broiled tomato
	½ baked sweet potato
2 medium rolls; 1 small pat butter	1 small cornmeal muffin; 2 small pats butter
½ grapefruit	Rice-raisin pudding made with ½ cup cooked rice, ½ cup milk, and 2 tablespoons raisins
Coffee or tea, if desired	Coffee or tea, if desired
Evening snack	**Evening snack**
1 small banana	12 grapes
¼ cup milk	Coffee or tea, if desired

From "Your Mild Sodium-Restricted Diet," American Heart Association, pp 25-26, 1969. © The American Heart Association. Used with permission.

have to perhaps one a week or one after every third meal. At other times, choose fruit.

- Pay attention to calories and read the labels on foods you buy in the store.
- Cut back on salt. Do not add salt at the table, avoid salty foods, and do not cook with salt.
- Eat smaller servings, and eat more slowly to give yourself time to feel full before you eat too much.

Eat several small meals instead of a few large ones.
• Avoid alcohol. It increases your appetite and in large amounts can raise your blood pressure.

The American Heart Association (AHA) has recently developed an eating plan (AHA diet) for healthy Americans. The plan includes the latest recommendations of medical scientists and provides a step-by-step guide to help you start a new lifestyle to lower your risks of heart attack and stroke. The plan is available free from your local Heart Association.

If you are overweight, choose whatever diet works best for you, but try to lose at least some of those extra pounds. Weight reduction is one of the most important things you can do on your own to lower your blood pressure. But remember: Weight loss helps to control your blood pressure and can decrease the number and amounts of drugs you need to take, but most patients with high blood pressure are not able to control it by weight loss alone. Such control might be possible, however, if you are only mildly hypertensive and can lose the weight and keep it off.

Check with your doctor before changing any of your medicines. Just because you are looking better and feeling good does not mean that your blood pressure has gone to levels that are low enough to be safe without medication.

In addition to limiting calories, be aware of special ingredients in your diet that can have either harmful or beneficial effects on your high blood pressure. These include salt, potassium, calcium, magnesium, cholesterol, fat, and alcohol. They are discussed below, as are the effects of cigarette smoking, exercise, and stress.

SALT

The most important thing you can do to help control your blood pressure besides losing weight may be to reduce your intake of salt. When doctors and patients refer to salt in the diet, they usually mean sodium, which is the part of salt that is most related to blood pressure. Studies have shown that groups of people around the world who eat a lot of salt have a higher rate of high blood pressure and groups of people who eat very little salt have a lower blood pressure. Animal studies also suggest a strong association between high blood pressure and salt intake. Dr. Walter Kempner used a sodium-free diet in the 1940s. It contained only rice and fruit and was effective in lowering blood pressure. Although some persons with high blood pressure do not respond very well to salt restriction, many others do.

Hypertensive people whose blood pressure can be lowered by salt restriction are called "salt sensitive." This type of high blood pressure is particularly common among diabetics, overweight individuals, elderly persons, and blacks. Since this is a common type of hypertension and salt restriction can do little or no harm, all persons with hypertension should limit their use of salt. Patients on diuretic therapy (water pills) for high blood pressure also gain additional benefit from restricting their intake of salt, since there can be an even better reduction in blood pressure and less loss of potassium.

A reduction of salt intake by half is usually adequate to improve blood pressure in hypertensive patients who are salt sensitive. To achieve this level of restricted sodium intake, you should use little or no salt at the table or in cooking, and do not eat processed foods or those in which salt can be tasted easily (ham, bacon, sausage, pickles, potato chips, salted nuts, etc.). Ethnic menus (e.g., soul food) that are high in salt should also be avoided or modified so that they become a delicacy rather than a routine part of the diet.

Table 4 shows a sample low-salt diet from the Chicago Heart Association. Table 5 gives you an idea of the kinds of foods that contain a lot of salt. You should try to avoid these foods unless they are labeled "low sodium."

Innovative approaches to diets should be studied to see if the sodium content can be reduced without changing the taste significantly. The black community should learn to "soulize" food without "sodiumizing" it.

TABLE 4. **Sample One-Day Menu for Mild Sodium (Salt) Restriction**
BREAKFAST

Amount	Food	Sodium (mg)
4 oz	Grapefruit juice	1
¾ oz	Puffed rice or wheat (without salt)	trace
8 oz	Skim milk	126
2 slices	Bread (white, rye or wheat)	292
2 tsp	Margarine	92
1 Tbsp	Jelly	trace
6 oz	Coffee	1
	Total*	513 mg

LUNCH

Amount	Food	Sodium (mg)
½ cup	Fruit	6
2 slices	Sandwich bread (white, rye or wheat)	292
2 oz	Chicken breast (roasted)	39
2 tsp	Mayonnaise	58
½	Tomato (3 to 4 slices, 3″ diameter)	3
4	Vanilla wafers	36
8 oz	Skim milk	126
	Total*	563 mg

DINNER

Amount	Food	Sodium (mg)
3 oz	Unsalted peanuts	15
4 oz	Halibut (broiled)	152
½ cup	Broccoli	28
2	Boiled potatoes with parsley	4
2 slices	Italian bread (3¼″ x 2½″)	118
3 tsp	Margarine	138
1 cup	Lettuce salad	trace
4 tsp	Oil	trace
2 tsp	Vinegar (cider or distilled)	trace
½ cup	Sherbet	5
6 oz	Coffee	1
	Total*	461 mg

SNACKS

Amount	Food	Sodium (mg)
1 cup	Unsalted popcorn	1
1	Whole carrot (7½" long)	34
8 oz	Skim milk	126
	Total*	161 mg
Daily TOTAL* (Breakfast, Lunch, Dinner, Snacks		1,698 mg

*Sodium content is calculated without added salt at table or in cooking.

From "Piecing Together the Sodium Puzzle," Chicago Heart Association, pp 13-15, 1979. Used with permission.

POTASSIUM

The role of potassium in high blood pressure has not been researched as thoroughly as the effects of sodium; however, studies suggest that high salt (sodium) intake is much more likely to cause high blood pressure if the amount of potassium in the diet is low.

Studies have shown that potassium intake in blacks is generally lower than in whites. It could be that poorer populations, such as the black urban poor, are unable to afford potassium-rich foods. New information suggests that some of the damage done to

TABLE 5. Examples of Foods and Snacks That Are Unusually High in Salt*

Bacon	Monosodium glutamate
Baking powder	(MSG)
Baking soda	Mustard
Beans	Olives
Bouillon (beef or chicken)	Pickles (dill or onion)
Bologna	Pig's feet (pickled)
Buttermilk (commercial)	Pizza
Canned meats (beef stew,	Pot pies
chili)	Potato chips
Canned soups	Pretzels
Canned vegetables	Salted nuts
Cheese	Salted peanuts
Cheeseburger	Saltines
Chitlins (pickled)	Sauerkraut
Fast foods	Sausage
Frozen foods	Seasonings†
Ham hock	Self-rising flour or meal
Hog maw (pickled)	Soda crackers
Hot dogs	Soy sauce
Instant grits	Steak sauces
Instant oatmeal	Tomato juice
Ketchup	TV dinners
Luncheon meats	

*These items, unless labeled "low sodium," should generally be avoided by persons who are trying to stay on a low-salt diet. The use of salt in cooking should also be avoided.

†Examples of seasonings that are high in sodium include Accent, celery salt, garlic salt, lemon pepper, onion salt, sea salt, and Season All.

the blood vessels of hypertensive persons might be made less severe by high-potassium diets.

Whether or not blood pressure can be brought down by taking extra potassium is not known for sure at this time; however, avoiding low potassium in the blood by eating a certain diet, taking drugs containing potassium, or using high blood pressure drugs that save potassium may be desirable for some people with high blood pressure. Foods high in potassium include mainly fresh fruits (and fruit juices) and vegetables. Bananas, raisins, oranges, grapefruit, potatoes, and spinach are high in potassium. For more detailed information on dietary sources of potassium, see Chapter 11 (Table 9).

You should be careful not to take extra potassium on your own unless you have first checked with your doctor, because it can be unsafe for some hypertensive patients with kidney damage or for those who are taking certain types of high blood pressure drugs.

CALCIUM

Patients with high blood pressure are sometimes found to have a low dietary intake of calcium. The low intake of calcium, however, is not necessarily a cause of the high blood pressure.

The body gets most of its calcium from dairy products such as milk and cheese. A low intake of calcium-rich foods can be a result of low income or stomach distress from milk (milk intolerance). Even though calcium intake may be low in some hypertensive individuals, a high dietary intake of calcium has not been proven to reduce blood pressure. Moreover, certain dairy products are rich in cholesterol and fats as well as calcium and can adversely affect the levels of fats and lipids in the blood.

OTHER MINERALS

Much less is known about how magnesium, zinc, and other minerals affect blood pressure. Low magnesium levels can cause weakness, twitching of the muscles, and irregular heartbeats, and zinc deficiency can cause abnormalities in the ability to taste or smell. Standard diuretic therapy can rarely cause a patient to become low in magnesium or zinc.

CHOLESTEROL AND FAT

There is a strong association between cholesterol and dietary fat and heart disease. In addition, recent studies have shown more high blood cholesterol levels among people with high blood pressure than those with normal blood pressure. Cholesterol, when present in high levels in the blood, can block the arteries to the heart and cause a heart attack. Your blood cholesterol can go up if you eat foods that contain a lot of cholesterol (eggs, cheese, cream, etc.) or too many highly saturated fat foods (animal fats, butter, meats, etc.), but you can also have high blood cholesterol because of genetic (inherited) factors.

A high blood cholesterol level does not by itself cause high blood pressure, but when it is present in a person with hypertension, the chance of having a heart attack is much greater because the cholesterol is more likely to deposit on the blood vessel walls and cause blockage. It is now considered optimal to have a blood cholesterol level below 200 mg/dl (milligrams per deciliter). Thus, you should know your cholesterol level and select foods that are low in cholesterol and saturated fats, such as low-fat dairy products, less red meats, and foods cooked with vegetable oils. This helps prevent any additional damage to your heart beyond what might have incurred from just the high blood pressure. Your doctor can order a simple blood test to check your cholesterol level. Table 6 provides information developed by the American Heart Association on the different kinds of fats in your diet.

ALCOHOL

It is now accepted that persons who drink excessive quantities of alcohol on a regular basis (more than two to three shots [4 ounces] of 100-proof whiskey, two glasses [16 ounces] of wine, or four cans [48 ounces] of beer a day) have increased risk of developing high blood pressure. Also, if high blood pressure is already present, heavy alcohol drinking will make it more difficult to control, even with medications. Thus, hypertensive patients are advised to keep their alcohol intake well below the limits indicated above.

CIGARETTE SMOKING

The public seems to be much more aware of cigarette smoking as a cause of lung cancer than as a cause of coronary artery disease (heart attacks). Cigarette smoking, high blood cholesterol and high blood pressure are the three big risk factors leading to heart attack, the number one cause of death in the United States. An even less well-known fact is that cigarette smoking also makes strokes more likely, as does high blood pressure. Therefore, people with high blood pressure are strongly urged not to smoke cigarettes if they wish to prevent a heart attack or stroke.

Today there are many books, programs and medications available to help you stop smoking. For further information on what is available, contact your doctor; your local hospital; the local chapter of the American Heart Association, American Cancer Society, or the American Lung Association; or programs of your national government or the World Health Organization (see Appendix III).

TABLE 6. Saturated Fats, Polyunsaturated Fats, and Cholesterol in Your Foods

Saturated Fats. This group of fats is found mostly in animal products. Saturated fat has a characteristically hard quality, such as the fat on beef. Saturated fats raise your blood cholesterol level more than other fats. Because of this, one of your objectives will be to reduce your saturated-fat intake.

Polyunsaturated Fats. These fats are found mostly in vegetable products and are characterized by a soft or liquid quality, such as corn oil. Since polyunsaturated fats lower cholesterol levels, one of your objectives will be to partially substitute polyunsaturated fat for the saturated fats you'll be eliminating.

Cholesterol. This fat-like substance is present only in animal products. Most Americans consume about 400 to 450 mg of cholesterol per day. Since dietary cholesterol raises blood cholesterol, your program should decrease your dietary cholesterol to less than 300 mg per day.

Foods contain a mixture of different kinds of fat. It is important to know the sources of these different fats. Foods high in saturated (bad) fats are mainly those of animal origin. For example, foods such as whole milk, cream, ice cream, cheese, butter, eggs, meat, and poultry are high in saturated fat. Palm and coconut oil are also highly saturated, as much as animal fats. Often, one of these fats is the primary fat in nondairy products (such as whipped topping) and commercially baked products, so be sure to read the food labels. Chocolate and many solid cooking fats are also saturated.

Adapted from "Eating for a Healthy Heart," American Heart Association, pp. 1-2, 1984. Used with permission.

EXERCISE

One can pick up almost any health book or manual and read that exercise is beneficial for whatever disease is being discussed. The popularity of exercise in the United States is phenomenal, but some caution is needed. Not all exercise is the same. Exercises such as running, swimming, and walking can lead to improved cardiovascular conditioning and generally are good for the patient with high blood pressure. With sufficient time, consistent aerobic exercise can reduce the resting pulse (heart rate) and blood pressure, so that medications for high blood pressure can sometimes be reduced or occasionally eliminated. Persons with high blood pressure must be careful to have exercise approved by their physician. The physician would usually want the blood pressure controlled before approving certain types or levels of exercise.

An exercise such as weight lifting is generally not advisable for most hypertensives. Very high levels of blood pressure can occur during this type of exercise.

STRESS

During the course of evaluating and treating a patient with high blood pressure, the physician may realize that stress plays a significant role in keeping the blood pressure elevated. Occupational stress can increase the likelihood of high blood pressure in susceptible persons. Racial, economic, and other societal stresses can also contribute to high rates of hypertension in different populations. Patients and physicians should be cautioned against believing that psychological stress is a major cause of high blood pressure in a specific individual. However, when emotional stress is felt to be contributing to high blood pressure, every effort should be made by the physician and patient to control it.

Techniques such as biofeedback and meditation are being studied and appear to be useful in helping to lower blood pressure levels in some patients. It is conceivable that spiritual healing, which may involve the "laying of hands" practiced by many pentecostal church groups, may also be useful in treating some patients with high blood pressure, especially if coupled with a strong positive attitude (e.g., "faith"). As with all treatments for high blood pressure, even when drugs are not used, a physician must be in charge to monitor the blood pressure on a regular basis and to ensure that no harm is done by any form of therapy and that medications are not discontinued prematurely.

SUMMARY

In this chapter we have discussed what you can do in conjunction with your physician to help control your blood pressure. We have included most of the forms of nondrug treatment for high blood pressure. We have tried to emphasize that even when drugs are used for high blood pressure, and they usually are, other measures are excellent additions to therapy. The things you can do may help to reduce the number of drugs, the amount of each drug, and the total cost of drugs necessary to control your blood pressure.

10

Drugs to Treat and Control High Blood Pressure: How Do They Work?

You can use the High Blood Pressure Drug Directory (Appendix I) to look up many high blood pressure drugs. The drugs are listed alphabetically by their brand or trade name. The name in parentheses is the generic name of the drug. Note that one drug may be manufactured by several companies that give it a different brand (trade) name. For example, labetalol is made by both Schering, which calls it Normodyne, and Glaxo, which calls it Trandate. This chapter will tell you what the high blood pressure drugs are and explain, in general, how they work. The next chapter will discuss the side effects of these drugs.

TREATMENT GOAL

The physician's primary goal when treating hypertension is to bring the diastolic blood pressure (bottom number) levels down to 90 mm Hg or less, and also often to reduce the systolic blood pressure (top number) to below 160 mm Hg, using the fewest drugs possible to help minimize side effects. To accomplish this, he or she can choose drugs that remove excess fluid from the body, that relax tightened (constricted) blood vessels, and/or that cause changes in certain parts of the nervous system.

Approximately half of all people with high blood pressure can control it with only one drug; three-fourths can control it through the use of, at most, two different blood pressure medicines; and nine out of ten can control the high blood pressure with three different drugs, or fewer.

TYPES OF DRUGS

The drugs used to treat high blood pressure belong, for the most part, to one of seven different classes. These are:

- diuretics
- beta blockers
- calcium channel blockers
- ACE inhibitors
- alpha blockers
- central agents
- vasodilators

Diuretics

Diuretics (water pills) are medicines that act directly on the kidneys to make you pass more urine.

They help rid the body of salt and water that may have accumulated in the blood, in the blood vessels, or in other parts of the body such as the areas around the feet, hands, or eyes. The decrease in salt and water reduces the volume of the blood and thus lowers blood pressure. For diuretics to be effective, you have to maintain a slightly lowered level of sodium in your body twenty-four hours a day. For this reason, you may still need to limit your salt intake while being careful to take your medicine exactly as prescribed. Diuretic drugs come in three general types: mild, strong, and potassium-saving.

Mild Diuretics. Examples of mild diuretics are hydrochlorothiazide, HydroDIURIL, Hygroton, Lozol, Naqua, Naturetin, and Zaroxolyn. The mild diuretics work as described above, acting directly on the kidneys to cause extra amounts of salt and water to come out in the urine.

Strong Diuretics. Strong diuretics act much more quickly than the mild diuretics, usually within an hour or two, but their effect does not last as long. They cause you to pass urine more quickly, but they are not necessarily more effective for lowering blood pressure than the mild diuretics. Examples of strong diuretics include Bumex and Lasix.

Potassium-sparing Diuretics. Potassium-sparing diuretics are generally mild, but unlike the other mild or strong diuretics, they do not cause potassium loss. Examples include Aldactone, Dyrenium, and Midamor. Potassium-sparing diuretics are often combined in the same tablet with a thiazide diuretic (Aldactazide, Dyazide, Maxzide, and Moduretic) to help prevent potassium deficiency in patients at risk of this disorder.

Beta Blockers

These drugs block structures in the body called beta receptors; hence, the name beta blockers. These receptors are located primarily in the heart, lungs, and blood vessel walls. Normally, beta receptors receive nerve and chemical signals that cause the heart to beat harder and faster or the blood vessels to constrict. When these receptors are blocked by a beta-blocking drug, the nerve message cannot get through to its destination. Blocking the receptors in the heart or blood vessel walls can keep the heart from beating too fast and can lead to an improvement in blood pressure. Blocking them in the lungs does not alter blood pressure but can cause or worsen asthma.

When high blood pressure patients take beta blockers, their pulse usually slows down. If it was 90 or 100 beats per minute before taking the medication, it may fall to 70 or 80; if it was 60 or 70 before, it may fall to 50 or 60. In general, it is not advisable to have the pulse rate fall much below 50 while you are awake. If your pulse is as high as 90 or 100, the doctor can usually tell that you are not taking enough of your beta blocker.

Types of Beta Blockers. There are many different beta blockers currently available in the United States and many more in other countries. All of them fall into one of several categories. "Cardioselective" beta blockers primarily affect the beta receptors that are in the heart. Examples include Kerlone, Lopressor, Sectral, and Tenormin. "Nonselective" beta blockers affect the beta receptors that are present in some other tissues (e.g., lungs, muscles, blood vessels) as well as those in the heart. Examples include Blocadren, Corgard, Inderal, Timolol, and Visken. Normodyne and Trandate are nonselective beta blockers, but they have another effect in addition to their nonselective beta blocker properties, called alpha block. Alpha receptors receive nerve and chemical signals that cause blood vessels to contract. When alpha receptors are blocked, the muscle tone of small arteries is relaxed, which widens their openings and decreases blood pressure. All of these beta blockers have roughly the same beneficial effect on blood pressure, but some people respond better to one type than another.

Besides improving blood pressure, beta blockers can also reduce chest pain, help prevent migraine headaches, and reduce your risk of having another heart attack if you have already had one.

Calcium Channel Blockers

Calcium is needed for the muscles of the heart and for blood vessels to contract. It seeps into muscle cells through pathways called calcium channels. Drugs that block these channels are called calcium channel blockers or calcium antagonists. If the calcium cannot enter, it cannot signal the muscle to contract. As a result, the muscles of the heart and blood vessels are relaxed by a calcium channel blocker. In many high blood pressure patients, there is excess constriction of the blood vessels. By acting directly at the site of the problem and helping to reduce the excess constriction, calcium blockers reduce blood pressure.

The calcium channel blockers currently available in the United States include Adalat, Calan, Cardene, Cardizem, DynaCirc, Isoptin, Plendil, and Procardia. All are effective in reducing blood pressure. As with the beta blockers, some people have fewer side effects or respond better to one calcium channel blocker than another.

A bonus effect of the calcium channel blockers is their improvement of some types of chest pain, such as angina, or special types of angina caused by spasms of the blood vessels of the heart.

ACE Inhibitors

ACE stands for angiotensin converting enzyme, and the drugs that inhibit this substance in the body are called ACE inhibitors. ACE inhibitors lower blood pressure mainly by preventing the body from making a powerful blood-vessel-tightening (or constricting) substance known as angiotensin II. Without this hormone, the blood vessels relax and blood pressure goes down. Examples of ACE inhibitors are Accupril, Altace, Capoten, Lotensin, Monopril, Prinivil, Vasotec, and Zestril.

Some, but not all ACE inhibitors are also indicated for treating heart failure, as well as high blood pressure. If you have both high blood pressure and heart failure, you may respond nicely to one of these drugs. In general, the ACE inhibitors are tolerated well with relatively few side effects. ACE inhibitors should not be taken by pregnant women.

Alpha Blockers

Alpha blockers are so named because they block structures in the body called alpha receptors. Alpha receptors, located mainly in the walls of blood vessels, receive nerve and chemical signals that cause blood vessels to constrict. When alpha receptors are blocked by an alpha-blocking drug, the blood vessels relax and blood pressure falls. Examples of alpha blockers are Cardura, Hytrin, and Minipress. Alpha blockers may also help to decrease the levels of fats and lipids in your blood.

Central Agents

Central agents work primarily in the lower part of the brain. They tell the nerves in the brain to release fewer chemical stimulants (e.g., norepinephrine), and when the level of these stimulants in the blood decreases, the blood vessels become more relaxed.

The four main central agents used for the treatment of high blood pressure are Aldomet, Catapres, Tenex, and Wytensin.

Vasodilators

Vasodilators act *directly* on the smooth muscles in the walls of blood vessels, causing them to relax (as opposed to some of the other types of drugs that relax the blood vessels indirectly by acting on nerves, etc.). Blood then flows more easily through the less constricted blood vessels, and blood pressure goes down. The two direct vasodilators used to treat high blood pressure are Apresoline and Loniten. Loniten is one of the most powerful blood pressure drugs that can be taken orally, but it is not used in the majority of patients because of its adverse effects.

Miscellaneous

Reserpine. Several good blood pressure drugs do not fit into one of the seven categories above. An example is reserpine (Serpasil), which works by depleting the body of the nerve stimulant norepinephrine. Reserpine is a major ingredient of Ser-Ap-Es, a combination of reserpine, Apresoline (hydralazine), and Esidrix (hydrochlorothiazide). Reserpine is often combined in the same tablet with a diuretic. Examples of this combination include Demi-Regroton, Diutensen-R, Diupres, Rauzide, Regroton, Renese-R, Salutensin, and Unipress.

Sympathetic Ganglion Blockers. The previously mentioned alpha and beta blockers act on the tiny (alpha and beta) receptors at nerve endings. There are also effective high blood pressure drugs that act on a larger part of the nerves, called the sympathetic ganglion. Ismelin is the classic drug of this type and was the only very powerful oral blood-pressure medicine available in the 1950s and 1960s. A more recently developed drug of this type, Hylorel, acts more quickly and has fewer and less severe side effects than Ismelin.

APPROACHES TO DRUG THERAPY

Stepped-Care Approach

Over the last five to fifteen years, most physicians have used a stepped-care approach in the use of medications for the treatment of high blood pressure. A beta blocker or diuretic is often chosen at first because these drugs have been used most in studies that have proven a long-term benefit to reduce the risk of stroke and other complications. The ACE inhibitors, calcium channel blockers, and alpha blockers can also be used for initial therapy, although they have not been well-tested to know whether they also will reduce stroke and other complications.

If control of blood pressure is not achieved with initial use of one of the types of drugs mentioned above, then a second drug (from a different class) is usually either added to or substituted for the initial drug. If blood pressure is still not controlled, then a third drug or a diuretic is then usually added if not already prescribed.

Individualized Approach

In some cases, your doctor may appropriately elect to use only one of the various classes of drugs. Through careful selection of the best drug for each particular patient, it may be possible to control that person's hypertension with only one drug (monotherapy) rather than with several. This is easier for many patients and helps to avoid both immediate and long-term side effects. In determining which drug to select for you, your physician will consider your age, race, other diseases that you may have, and the costs and potential side effects of the drug.

In the past five years, the availability of new medications has led many physicians to modify the stepped-care approach and individualize therapy for each patient. The objective of all treatment programs is to achieve the most effective treatment at the lowest cost and with the fewest drug-related side effects.

INTERACTIONS OF BLOOD PRESSURE MEDICINES WITH OTHER DRUGS

Patients often ask if there are any medicines they should not take when they are on high blood pressure drugs. We have already mentioned that some cold remedies contain pseudoephedrine, phenylpropanolamine, or phenylephrine, which can raise blood pressure. A small amount of alcohol usually does not react with blood pressure medicines, but heavy alcohol intake can lead to excess loss of fluid from your body (dehydration) if you are also taking a diuretic.

Certain drugs, when combined with specific blood pressure medicines, can lead to potentially dangerous reactions. But this does not mean that these drugs can never be taken together—you may be doing very well on the combination and should continue. Some of these drugs, the blood pressure medicines involved, and the possible reactions are listed in Table 7.

TABLE 7. Possible Reactions Caused by Combining High Blood Pressure Medication with Other Drugs*

Non-High-Blood-Pressure Drug	Usual Clinical Use	High Blood Pressure Drug	Possible Danger
Parnate†	Depression	Hylorel, Ismelin	Taking Parnate could cause the high blood pressure drug to lose its effect.
Insulin	Diabetes	Beta blockers, especially Corgard, Inderal, Levacor, Timolol, or Visken	An insulin reaction with low blood sugar can go unrecognized or last much longer than usual.
Lithium carbonate	Manic depression	Thiazide diuretics	Therapy with thiazide-type diuretics can cause the blood level of lithium to rise to toxic levels.
Potassium supplements	Low blood potassium	Potassium-saving diuretics‡	The blood level of potassium can sometimes become too high, causing the heart to stop.

TABLE 7. Possible Reactions Caused by Combining High Blood Pressure Medication with Other Drugs* (continued)

Non-High-Blood-Pressure Drug	Usual Clinical Use	High Blood Pressure Drug	Possible Danger
Dilantin	Seizures	Lasix	Dilantin can reduce the effectiveness of Lasix.
Nonsteroidal anti-inflammatory agents**	Arthritis	Lasix	The arthritis drugs can reduce the effectiveness of the diuretic so that the dose of Lasix might need to be increased.
		Beta blockers, ACE inhibitors	The arthritis drugs can sometimes reduce the blood pressure lowering effect of the beta blockers or ACE inhibitors.
Tricyclic antidepressants††	Depression	Aldomet, Catapres, Hylorel, Ismelin, Reserpine	Taking these antidepressant drugs can interfere with the blood pressure lowering effect of the drugs listed.
Digoxin	Heart problems	Calan, Isoptin	The dosage of digoxin may need to be reduced in certain cases to avoid arrhythmias.

TABLE 7. Possible Reactions Caused by Combining High Blood Pressure Medication with Other Drugs* (continued)

Non-High-Blood-Pressure Drug	Usual Clinical Use	High Blood Pressure Drug	Possible Danger
Cyclosporine	Organ transplants	Calcium channel blockers, except Procardia	Increase in the blood level and toxicity of cyclosporine.

*For a more complete listing of possible interactions of each of these drugs with other drugs, please refer to either the *Physician's Desk Reference (PDR)* or the information about a particular drug available from your pharmacist.

†Patients taking this type of drug can also experience severe elevation of blood pressure if they eat significant amounts of food that contain a substance called tyramine. Examples of foods particularly high in tyramine include cheddar cheese, Gruyere cheese, pickled herring, chianti wine, and chicken livers.

‡Including Aldactazide, Aldactone, Dyazide, Maxzide, Midamor, and Moduretic.

**Such as Indocin and possibly also Anaprox, Clinoril, Feldene, Meclomen, Motrin, Nalfon, Naprosyn, and Tolectin.

††A few examples include Aventyl, Elavil, Norpramin, Pertofrane, Presamine, Sinequan, Tofranil, and Vivactil

11

What Are Common Side Effects of High Blood Pressure Drugs?

DRUG SIDE EFFECTS

All drugs, including aspirin and Tylenol, have some unwanted (adverse) side effects. Many of the drugs and their potential side effects are listed in the *Physician's Desk Reference (PDR)*, a listing of drugs compiled by many pharmaceutical firms. Your doctor's goal is to choose a drug that is effective for your particular case of high blood pressure, and one that has few side effects for you.

Side effects from high blood pressure drugs are difficult for the physician to evaluate because they are often symptoms that you may have had before taking the drug. For example, 10 to 20 percent of people *not* taking high blood pressure drugs experience fatigue, headache, dizziness, constipation, sexual dysfunction, or periods of mild depression. The notable feature of a drug-related side effect is that it begins after you start taking the drug and usually goes away when your doctor reduces the amount of the drug or switches you to different type of therapy.

The blood pressure drugs available in the 1950s and early 1960s were associated with more side effects, and it was necessary for some patients to live with severe side effects as a trade-off to reduce their risk of stroke. In the 1990s, however, fewer people develop side effects from the newer blood pressure drugs. Unfortunately, side effects continue to occur, in as few as one in every twenty to as many as one in every four patients taking blood pressure medications, depending on the drug used. Some of the common bothersome side effects include muscle weakness, headaches, and insomnia. Table 8 gives examples of many of the bothersome side effects, and the antihypertensive drugs most likely to cause them.

If you have or develop any side effects, don't be shy—tell your doctor so that he or she can evaluate the symptoms and determine if any change in your medicine is needed.

Muscle Weakness

Hypokalemia, a low level of potassium in your blood, is a condition that can be caused by the use of diuretics such as hydrochlorothiazide, Hygroton, Lasix, Bumex, Lozol, or Zaroxolyn. These diuretics eliminate extra salt and water through your kidneys, but they can also cause an unwanted loss of potassium.

Your potassium level can only be determined by a blood test. Usually this test and other blood tests (e.g., chemistries or electrolytes) are done before

TABLE 8. Side Effects of High Blood Pressure Drugs*

Brand or Trade Name	Generic Name	Examples of Bothersome Side Effects
Accupril	quinapril	cough, rash
Adalat	nifedipine	headache, swelling of legs
Aldomet	methyldopa	sleepiness, impotence, hepatitis
Altace	ramipril	cough, rash
Apresoline	hydralazine	headaches, pounding heart, lupus erythematosus
Blocadren	timolol	fatigue, shortness of breath
Bumex	bumetanide	weak muscles, frequent urination, gout
Calan	verapamil	constipation, dizziness
Capoten	captopril	cough, rash
Cardene	nicardipine	headache, swelling of legs
Cardizem	diltiazem	headache, dizziness
Cardura	doxazosin	dizziness
Catapres	clonidine	sleepiness, dry mouth
Corgard	nadalol	fatigue, shortness of breath, numb hands
Dyazide	†	frequent urination, gout
DynaCirc	isradipine	headache, swelling of legs
Esidrix	hydrochlorothiazide	weak muscles, frequent urination, gout
Hygroton	chlorthalidone	weak muscles, frequent urination, gout
Hylorel	guanadrel	dizziness, passing out
Hytrin	terazosin	dizziness

TABLE 8. **Side Effects of High Blood Pressure Drugs*** (continued)

Brand or Trade Name	Generic Name	Examples of Bothersome Side Effects
Inderal	propranolol	fatigue, shortness of breath, sleep disturbance, numb hands
Ismelin	guanethidine	dizziness, passing out, impotence
Isoptin	verapamil	constipation, dizziness
Kerlone	betaxolol	fatigue, shortness of breath, numb hands
Lasix	furosemide	weak muscles, frequent urination, gout
Levatol	penbutalol	fatigue, shortness of breath, numb hands
Loniten	minoxidil	swelling of legs, excess hair growth
Lopressor	metoprolol	fatigue, sleep disturbance
Lotensin	benazepril	cough, rash
Lozol	metolazone	weak muscles, frequent urination, gout
Maxzide	†	frequent urination, gout
Minipress	prazosin	dizziness, irregular heartbeats
Monopril	fosinopril	cough, rash
Naturetin	bendroflumethiazide	weak muscles, frequent urination, gout
Normodyne	labetalol	fatigue, dizziness, tingling scalp
Norvasc	amlodipine	headache, swelling of legs
Plendil	felodipine	headache, swelling of legs
Prinivil	lisinopril	cough, rash
Procardia	nifedipine	headache, swelling of legs

TABLE 8. Side Effects of High Blood Pressure Drugs* (continued)

Brand or Trade Name	Generic Name	Examples of Bothersome Side Effects
Reserpine	reserpine	listlessness, depression
Tenex	guanfacine	sleepiness, dry mouth
Tenormin	atenolol	fatigue, dizziness
Trandate	labetalol	fatigue, dizziness, tingling scalp
Vasotec	enalapril	cough, rash
Verelan	verapamil	constipation, dizziness
Visken	pindolol	fatigue, odd dreams
Wytensin	guanabenz	sleepiness, dry mouth
Zaroxolyn	metolazone	weak muscles, frequent urination, gout
Zestril	lisinopril	cough, rash

*For a much more complete listing of side effects of each of these drugs, please refer to either the *Physician's Desk Reference (PDR)* or the package insert for a particular drug available at your pharmacy.

†A "combination" type blood pressure drug (diuretic) containing both hydrochlorothiazide and triamterene.

TABLE 9. Examples of Food Rich in Potassium

Item	Amount	Milliequivalents of Potassium	Calories	Milligrams of Sodium
Prune juice*	1 glass†	15.1	193	5
Tomato juice	1 glass	13.7	48	480
Cantaloupe	One-half	12.8	60	24
Potato (baked)	One medium	12.8	95	4
Grapefruit juice	1 glass	11.8	108	3
Orange juice	1 glass	10.7	120	3
Milk (skim)	1 glass	10.5	89	128
Raisins	⅓ cup	10.4	153	14
Milk (whole)	1 glass	9.5	150	120
Banana	One (6″)	9.5	85	1
Pineapple juice	1 glass	9.2	128	<1
Tomato	One medium	8.1	29	5
Orange	One medium	8.0	71	2
Pear	One medium	6.7	122	4
Apple juice	1 glass	6.2	120	8
Peach	One medium	5.2	38	1
Apple	One medium	4.2	87	1
Grapefruit	One-half	3.5	41	1
Black coffee	1 cup	2.2	2	1

*All juice values are as canned, unsweetened

†1 glass = 8 ounces

you begin blood pressure therapy. The normal serum potassium level is about 4.5, with a range between 3.5 and 5.2 mEq/L (milliequivalents per liter). In most patients, diuretic therapy will cause the blood potassium level to fall to between 3.5 and 4.0 mEq/L. About one in every four patients, however, can develop hypokalemia, with a potassium level below 3.5.

"Mild" hypokalemia (blood potassium levels between 3.0 and 3.5) usually has no symptoms and can be treated with medicines that contain potassium, such as Kay Ciel elixir, K-Dur, K-Lor, K-Lyte, Kaon-Cl, Kato, Kaochlor, Slow-K, Micro-K, or combination diuretics with a special ingredient that holds onto potassium.

A low level of blood potassium can also be treated by increasing the amount of potassium in your diet, although this requires that you eat or drink fairly large amounts of certain things. Potassium-rich foods (listed in Table 9) include fruits and juices. The very best types of foods to eat to add extra potassium to your diet should contain a lot of potassium but few calories and not much salt (sodium). Table 9 shows why orange juice, bananas, and grapefruit juice are often recommended. Tomato juice and milk are good sources of potassium but contain too much sodium. Prune juice and raisins are high in potassium but contain many calories.

The amount of potassium in the diet of normal Americans ranges from 30 to 80 milliequivalents a day (1170 to 3120 milligrams a day). People with mild hypokalemia may need as much as 40 to 60 milliequivalents of extra potassium daily. Salt substitutes, which you can buy at the grocery store, can also be useful and provide about 50 to 65 milliequivalents of potassium per teaspoon. Some of the brands are Adolphs Salt Substitute, Co-Salt, Diasol, Featherweight Seasoned Salt Substitute, Neocurtasal, and Nu-Salt. Another excellent but little-known dietary source of potassium is cream of tartar, a relatively tasty condiment.

Do not suddenly start eating high-potassium foods or change to a salt substitute. Check with your doctor first because extra amounts of dietary potassium can be very dangerous for high blood pressure patients with certain other problems, such as kidney failure.

"Severe" hypokalemia (serum potassium levels below 3) occurs in about one out of every twenty patients who take relatively high dosages of diuretics. It can cause no symptoms at all or it can be associated with profound muscle weakness such that you barely have the strength in your legs to walk up a hill, climb stairs, or get up out of a chair, or enough strength in your arms to brush your hair or lift a fork. Joggers, weight lifters, and people in jobs requiring considerable physical labor may experience bad muscle pains after exertion. Some people also get odd tingly feelings (paresthesias) in their arms and legs, but these are unusual unless there is some muscle weakness as well. (Tingling of the fingers or toes can also be caused by some of the beta blockers.) Left untreated, severe hypokalemia can cause irregular heartbeats, which can be dangerous. These can occur in anybody, but are especially likely in persons who are also taking the heart medicine digoxin

(Lanoxin). Severe hypokalemia is treated with a high-potassium diet, potassium supplements, or a reduction of the dosage of your diuretic, when feasible. It may also be an indication to change to a type of diuretic that saves rather than loses potassium. The potassium-saving diuretics include Aldactazide, Aldactone, Dyazide, Maxzide, Midamor, and Moduretic.

Sleepiness

Certain high blood pressure drugs that act in your brain mainly to calm down the nerve traffic tend to make you sleepy. Those medicines that are most likely to cause sleepiness are Aldomet, Catapres, Tenex, and Wytensin. If you have just started taking one of these drugs and feel sleepy all of the time, be extra careful about driving, and try not to fall asleep on the job. This effect is often most apparent when first starting the medicine and tends to get better after a week or two.

Diuretics, calcium channel blockers, ACE inhibitors, and vasodilators rarely, if ever, cause sleepiness.

Fatigue

The most common causes of fatigue are overwork, depression, not getting enough restful sleep, and being under stress. However, some blood pressure medicines can cause fatigue that differs from the sleepiness discussed above. Very active people may notice that they feel worn out at the end of the day or while exercising; other people may think that they are just getting old and cannot do as much or walk as far as they used to. Some of the blood pressure drugs, such as the beta blockers, can cause this effect, including Blocadren, Corgard, Inderal, Kerlone, Levacor, Lopressor, Normodyne, Sectral, Tenormin, Toprol XL, and Trandate. Many older patients feel "born again" when their dosage of beta blockers is reduced, or they change to other drugs that are equally effective. Beta blockers are especially good at helping angina and preventing recurrence of heart attack, but chest pain or irregular heartbeats can occur if the beta blocker is discontinued abruptly or if the dosage is reduced too rapidly. You should never stop taking or reduce the dosage of your beta blocker on your own; check with your doctor first.

As mentioned earlier, fatigue can also occur in patients with a low level of potassium resulting from diuretic therapy. ACE inhibitors, calcium channel blockers, and vasodilators are the classes of drugs that are least likely to cause fatigue.

Dizziness

Dizziness is one of the most common reasons people have for visiting the doctor and its cause is usually not determined. One cause of dizziness is an imbalance of fluids in the inner-ear canals, especially if the dizziness is accompanied by ringing in the ears, nausea, or a feeling that the room is spinning around. Another type of dizziness, not related to the ear canals, can be caused either by high blood pressure or by a sharp drop in blood pressure, which can be caused by some medications. Dizziness from high blood pressure is usually a vague feeling of giddiness and imbalance with a sense of unsteadiness centered in your head. It often occurs after getting up suddenly or rising from a squatting position. Light-headedness caused by a drop in blood pressure is more a feeling that you are about to faint. You may see spots in front of your eyes, such as can occur when you get up too suddenly in the morning.

If your blood pressure drops too much when you stand up, the condition is called orthostatic hypotension. It can occur naturally in older people, or it can be caused by certain drugs. The worst offender is Ismelin, but it can also be caused by Aldomet, Cardura, Catapres, Hylorel, Hytrin, Minipress, Normodyne, Trandate, or almost any of the high blood pressure drugs, especially if you start them in addition to diuretic therapy. Minipress can cause marked dizziness and dropping of blood pressure when it is first started, but this effect usually becomes less apparent as therapy continues.

Depression

Depression is fairly common among both men and women and its cause is usually not apparent. It can, however, be associated with a variety of medications for high blood pressure. In the past, reserpine was the antihypertensive drug most often accused of causing depression. Drugs containing reserpine are Demi-Regroton, Diutensin-R, Diupres, Rauzide, Renese-R, Salutensin, Ser-Ap-Es, and Unipres. Depression is most likely to occur if dosages of reserpine exceed 0.125 mg daily; it is much less frequent with the lower dosages currently recommended.

Depression can occur with other antihypertensive drugs, including the beta blockers and centrally acting agents (Aldomet, Catapres, Tenex, Wytensin). One study noted that 23 percent of patients on beta blockers were also receiving antidepressant drugs. Drug-related depression is most unusual with the use of ACE inhibitors, alpha blockers, or calcium channel blockers.

Headaches

Headaches are not a good indication of high blood pressure in most people since they are fairly common even in people whose blood pressure is normal. Many headaches are related to tension or spasms of the neck muscles. The blood pressure drug that is most likely to provoke headaches is Apresoline; it directly dilates, or widens, the blood vessels.

Insomnia

Certain blood pressure medications may cause you to wake up repeatedly throughout the night and recall dreams that may be vivid or frightening.

The drugs most likely to interfere with sleep are the beta blockers, particularly high dosages of Inderal (320 mg a day or more) or Visken (40 mg a day or more). Insomnia and abnormal dreaming can often be improved by switching to a beta blocker that does not enter the brain as much, such as Tenormin.

Skin Rash

Many rashes are caused by pimples, heat, infection, or contact with an irritant such as poison ivy, a new perfume, or a new piece of clothing colored with chemical dyes. However, there are also certain types of blood pressure drugs that can cause rashes due to an allergy to the drug. Approximately one out of every one hundred to five hundred patients who use the thiazide diuretic drugs will develop a rash. This particular rash is often photosensitive; it breaks out after exposure to sunlight (e.g., after a trip to the beach).

The ACE inhibitors cause rashes in approximately one of every twenty-five to one hundred patients. These rashes, which often occur during the first few weeks after starting the drug, may be reddish eruptions on various parts of the body. In very rare circumstances, a scaly rash that looks like psoriasis will occur in patients receiving beta blockers. Rashes can also occur with the calcium channel blockers.

Impotence and Other Sexual Problems

Impotence is an inability to carry out normal sexual function. It can be psychological or organic, but the most common causes are either psychological or related to excess alcohol intake. Some blood pressure medications interfere with sexual function. They can cause men to lose interest in sex or have difficulty in obtaining or maintaining an erection. This is most commonly seen with Aldomet, but sexual impotence can also result from any other antihypertensive drugs, including the diuretics and beta blockers. Ismelin can cause men to ejaculate backwards so that no semen comes out. Blood pressure drugs do not usually cause premature ejaculation (the tendency for the male to ejaculate during foreplay or after the first few seconds of vaginal entry).

Some blood pressure medications (e.g., beta blockers) also cause sexual problems in women, such as a decrease in the desire for sex (libido), muscle spasms of the vagina (vaginismus), or poor lubrication.

Blood pressure drugs that rarely, if ever, cause sexual problems include Apresoline, the ACE inhibitors, and the calcium channel blockers.

Fortunately, when impotence is a side effect of high blood pressure medications, it will usually disappear when the drug is stopped or the dosage is reduced.

Swelling of the Breasts

A swelling of one or both breasts can occur in men or women. The condition is called gynecomastia. The swelling typically occurs just under the nipple, but can involve the entire breast area. Sometimes the breasts will feel tender and on occasion, there may be secretion of milk (lactation) from the nipple.

Gynecomastia is an infrequent side effect of any of the blood pressure drugs but occurs most with the use of Aldomet, Aldactazide, and Aldactone. It is also reported with the calcium channel blockers. Aldomet causes an increase in the blood levels of the milk-secreting hormone prolactin, but the breast swelling and tenderness, as well as the lactation, if present, typically disappear completely within a week or so of stopping the drug. Several non-blood-pressure drugs can also cause gynecomastia (e.g., heart pills such as digoxin [Lanoxin]).

Dry Mouth

Most of the diuretics, if they are effective, will cause some dryness of the mouth. This is usually not very bothersome, although you will want to drink more water. Catapres, Tenex, and Wytensin, however, tend to dry the mouth more severely, so this can become an aggravating side effect.

Leg and Muscle Cramps

Leg cramps are common and they tend to occur at night. They are not necessarily related to poor circulation. Nocturnal (nighttime) leg cramps are especially common in hypertensive patients who also have diabetes, and can be very painful. Nocturnal leg cramps are not well understood, but often are improved through therapy with quinine or Benadryl.

Leg cramps sometimes occur after first starting diuretics, especially when the diuretics have a strong effect, as they do in patients with swelling (edema) of the legs. The cramps are caused by the drawing out of salt and water from the leg muscles and usually subside after the first three or four days of therapy.

Another type of leg cramp can be caused by claudication. Claudication, pain felt in the calves of the legs when you are walking, can be the result of a blockage of the vessels supplying blood to the leg muscles; however, it is not usually caused by blood pressure medication.

Swelling of the Legs

Some blood pressure medicines cause the kidneys to retain salt and water, exactly the opposite effect of a diuretic. Swelling of the legs is a particular problem of Loniten, which can cause retention of 5 to 10 pounds of body fluid during the first week of therapy. The drug must usually be administered concomitantly with a diuretic to prevent fluid retention. The feet, ankles, and legs can swell, making shoes fit poorly. Rarely, the hands can also swell, and wedding rings sometimes have to be cut. Aldomet can also cause this swelling, but to a lesser degree than Loniten. Swelling of the legs can also occur during therapy with some of the calcium channel blockers such as Adalat, DynaCirc, Norvasc, or Plendil.

Breathing Trouble

Many patients with high blood pressure have trouble breathing, but it is usually the result of lung disease from emphysema or asthma associated with past cigarette smoking. High blood pressure does not damage the lungs or cause breathing trouble unless the heart fails. If the heart has been damaged, you may experience breathing trouble when you are resting flat at night. This particular breathing problem usually improves if you sit up for five or ten minutes. Doctors call it PND, or paroxysmal nocturnal dyspnea, when patients wake up suddenly short of breath at night.

Certain blood pressure drugs, especially the beta blockers, can sometimes cause more shortness of breath or attacks of asthma if you are already predisposed to this problem. This can be the result of blocking the beta receptors in the lung (see Chapter 10). The worst offenders are Blocadren, Corgard, Inderal, Levacor, and Timolol. Kerlone, Lopressor, Tenormin, and Visken are beta blockers less likely to cause shortness of breath. Reserpine is a blood pressure drug that sometimes causes a minor but aggravating sort of troubled breathing because of a stuffy nose.

Cough

A very peculiar adverse effect of the ACE inhibitors is the occurrence of an aggravating dry cough without other signs of an upper respiratory infection. The cough is relatively common, occurring in as many as one out of every 7 to 10 patients treated with ACE inhibitors. There is nothing wrong with the lungs and the cough usually disappears completely within a few days of stopping the drug. It doesn't do any good to change to a different type of ACE inhibitor, although sometimes the cough improves following a decrease in dosage of the drug.

Gout

Diuretics increase the risk of developing a very painful type of arthritis called gout. Gout usually causes redness and painful swelling of the big toe, but it can also attack elsewhere in the foot or in the knee, hip, or shoulder. The diuretics (especially thiazide diuretics) tend to promote gout by raising the blood level of a substance called uric acid. When the level of uric acid becomes too high, it can lead to the formation of sharp uric acid crystals that can settle in a joint and cause pain.

The level of uric acid can usually be controlled by drugs that help eliminate it through the kidneys (Benemid or probenecid) or that cause the body to make less of it (Zyloprim or allopurinol). A physician may also elect to switch from diuretic therapy to other blood pressure medicines, since only the diuretics tend to cause gout.

High Blood Cholesterol

Certain blood pressure drugs, primarily the diuretics and beta blockers, can cause an increase in the blood level of fats, such as cholesterol and triglycerides. This 6 to 15 percent increase tends to occur mainly in the first year of treatment, and is worrisome because it can potentially increase the risk of cardiac problems such as heart attack. Patients being treated with diuretics or beta blockers should reduce their intake of calories and cholesterol, especially if they have a family history of heart disease. Certain beta blockers (e.g., Visken) and diuretics (Aldactone and low dosages of Lozol) have been shown not to cause these problems. In addition, alpha blockers do not increase (and sometimes actually decrease) the levels of fats and lipids in your blood. ACE inhibitors and calcium channel blockers have no adverse effects on blood lipids.

Irregular Heartbeats

Irregular or "skippy" heartbeats occur when you suddenly feel one or more flip-flops of your heart. They usually last for just a few seconds but can continue for much longer periods of time. Doctors usually call these irregular beats "palpitations," a term that means you can sense or feel the skipped beats. Many people have skip beats and never know it. However, they can be detected by an electrocardiogram (or Holter monitor) and sometimes by just feeling the pulse.

Skippy heartbeats are not always bad. They often occur in people who drink too much coffee or alcohol. They can also occur if you are overworked and fatigued, during extreme excitement, or if you are very angry about something. It is perfectly normal for the heart to beat hard and thump in your chest when you are excited or stimulated (as during intercourse, physical exercise, or a close call on the expressway), but it should not skip beats very often when you are resting.

Some people have skippy heartbeats because of an inadequate flow of blood from the coronary arteries to the heart. This can occur when cholesterol and other fats in the blood accumulate in the walls of the coronary arteries and make them too narrow.

Irregular beats are also more common in high blood pressure patients if the heart has become enlarged. A current area of controversy among high blood pressure experts is whether skipped beats are sometimes caused by treatment with diuretic drugs. Some research has indicated that the loss of minerals like potassium or magnesium, for example, can result from use of these diuretics and may account for the occurrence of irregular heartbeats, particularly if you have already developed an enlarged heart from high blood pressure or if you have coronary artery disease.

Concern about the risks of skippy heartbeats from the use of diuretics that do not save potassium has led some physicians to reduce the usual dosage of diuretics when possible and sometimes to begin treatment with other kinds of drugs. However, the risk of developing too much potassium loss or skip beats is reduced markedly with the much lower doses of diuretics recommended currently.

Hepatitis

Most cases of hepatitis are due to a viral infection that causes damage to the liver, but hepatitis can also occur because of an allergic reaction that is a side effect of antihypertensive therapy. Aldomet, for example, can sometimes cause a liver reaction during the first two to three months of therapy. There are usually no symptoms or evidence of a viral infection, except that the blood liver test called SGOT will be positive. The hepatitis generally clears up within a few weeks of stopping the drug. If you have ever had hepatitis caused by Aldomet, remember that you are sensitive or allergic to it, and be sure not to take it again because the reaction can be worse the second time around.

Lupus Erythematosus

Lupus erythematosus is a disease caused by a person producing antibodies (autoantibodies) that attack his or her own tissues. It occurs most often in young women and usually begins with a skin rash and painful joints. Rarely, very high dosages (i.e., 300 to 400 mg daily) of Apresoline can cause it, but it usually clears up when the medicine is stopped.

LIVING WELL WITH DRUG THERAPY

Twenty-five years ago, hypertensive patients often faced a difficult choice: Indure unwanted side effects or suffer from uncontrolled high blood pressure. Today, in the vast majority of cases, such a choice is unnecessary. By carefully selecting from the many drugs now available, your physician can tailor drug treatment to your particular needs so you can control your blood pressure and maintain a high quality of life.

12

What If I Have High Blood Pressure and Other Diseases?

It is possible that you may suffer from another disease as well as high blood pressure, especially if you are older. In some cases, the combined effects of high blood pressure and other diseases can increase the rate of damage to the body and put certain medications "off limits" because of their undesirable side effects. This chapter will discuss the things that you should keep in mind if you have high blood pressure and you also suffer from heart failure, heart disease, heartbeat irregularities, circulation problems, diabetes, asthma, emphysema, or gout.

HEART FAILURE

Heart failure can be a complication of severe or uncontrolled high blood pressure. Heart failure can also be caused by a viral infection, rheumatic heart disease, leaky heart valves, or multiple heart attacks. If you have poorly controlled heart failure and high blood pressure, you would usually not want to take drugs such as the beta blockers or the calcium channel blocker verapamil, which reduce the force of the heart's pumping action. A better choice might be an ACE inhibitor that reduces your blood pressure by dilating the blood vessels without having a negative effect on the heart. A diuretic is also a good choice for high blood pressure if heart failure exists.

HEART DISEASE

If untreated for many years, high blood pressure can lead to narrowing and stiffening of the arteries (arteriosclerosis) and a decrease in the supply of blood to the heart. This reduced blood flow decreases the supply of oxygen to the heart muscle and can produce angina (chest pain felt on exertion, caused by starving the heart muscle of proper nutrition) or heart attack (death of the heart muscle from lack of nutrition). Fatty accumulations inside the arteries (atherosclerosis) can worsen the effects of arteriosclerosis, increasing the damage to the heart.

Thiazide diuretics and some of the beta blockers can sometimes cause an increase in the levels of fat in the blood, but for many people, that increase does not produce any observable effect for many years. For this reason, if laboratory tests show that you have high levels of fat (cholesterol or triglycerides) in your blood, you may need to be on a special diet, take a lower dosage of the diuretic, or change from a diuretic to one of the other high blood pressure medications available that does not raise cholesterol (i.e., calcium channel blocker, alpha blocker, or ACE inhibitor). On the other hand, calcium channel blockers, some beta blockers, and nitrates may be very useful in heart disease (coronary disease) when present with high blood pressure.

HEARTBEAT IRREGULARITIES

High blood pressure can also lead to irregular heartbeats, known as arrhythmias. The likelihood of this happening increases if the amount of potassium in your blood decreases. For this reason, it is sometimes helpful to take extra potassium or special water pills that hold onto potassium (generally, water pills decrease the amount of potassium in your blood) or to use blood pressure drugs—such as ACE inhibitors, calcium channel antagonists, alpha blockers, or beta blockers—that do not decrease the levels of potassium in the blood.

CIRCULATION PROBLEMS

Patients with circulation problems may complain of cold feet and hands because of decreased blood flow. If they also have high blood pressure they should monitor their feet or hand symptoms carefully since some, but not all, of the beta blockers can cause narrowing of the blood vessels, which decreases blood flow even more.

DIABETES

One of the long-term effects of untreated hypertension is the narrowing and stiffening of blood vessels (including those in the eye), which increase the likelihood that they might burst and hemorrhage. Since diabetes can lead to abnormal growth in the blood vessels of the eye, the additive effect of diabetes to hypertension greatly increases the likelihood of developing eye problems and possibly blindness. Similarly, the combination of diabetes and high blood pressure increases the rate of damage to the kidneys and the likelihood of kidney failure.

You can do much to avoid such damage by controlling your high blood pressure with medications and watching your diet and insulin requirements. But you might not want to take a beta blocker to control your high blood pressure if you are a brittle (hard to treat) diabetic with blood sugar levels that bounce around a lot, since this class of drugs could hide some of the signs of low blood sugar or bring out an underlying tendency to have diabetes. Low blood sugar causes rapid beating of the heart, but beta blockers act to slow the heart. For this reason, a diabetic who is taking beta blockers might not be able to detect an insulin reaction, which is caused by dangerously low levels of blood sugar.

Thiazide diuretics must be used with caution in patients with borderline diabetes, since these drugs can raise the level of blood sugar or produce diabetes. New studies are suggesting that certain drugs used to treat high blood pressure may help protect the kidney in diabetes. The calcium channel blockers and ACE inhibitors are two classes of drugs that seem to be promising in this area.

ASTHMA, BRONCHITIS, AND EMPHYSEMA

Asthma, bronchitis, and emphysema are all associated with the narrowing of the air passages in the lungs and the resultant difficulty in breathing. In some cases, the narrowing can be reversed by the use of certain medications such as steroids (e.g., prednisone). But these same medications can aggravate high blood pressure by increasing the narrowing of the arteries and/or causing salt retention.

Similarly, some drugs that lower blood pressure can increase breathing difficulties. Most beta blockers, for example, narrow the air passages in the lungs. High blood pressure drugs that cause sleepiness must also be used with caution in patients with severe lung problems, because oversedation could aggravate the ability to breathe fully.

GOUT

Gout, a painful form of arthritis, is the result of uric acid accumulating in the joints. If you have gout and high blood pressure, you might not want to take a thiazide diuretic to treat the high blood pressure, since these water pills can increase the levels of uric acid in the blood.

Gout is associated with a high protein or alcohol intake and, usually, with being overweight. Since excess weight and heavy drinking also raise your blood pressure, you can expect both gout and blood pressure to improve if you lose weight and decrease your alcohol intake.

SUMMARY

If you suffer from other diseases as well as high blood pressure, your doctor will want to monitor your condition carefully and be certain that medication prescribed for one disease does not cause side effects that could worsen the symptoms of the other disease. You should keep your doctor fully informed about your symptoms and any prescription or over-the-counter medications you might be taking.

13

Taking Your Blood Pressure Medicines

High blood pressure is a disease that has few symptoms. For example, you don't feel sick so the motivation to keep taking medicines is less than, for instance, a chest infection. Compliance to the prescription, that is, taking the correct amount of medicine at the correct time for the right length of time, is extremely important. A medicine is only effective if it is taken correctly.

Why is taking your medicine as directed (compliance) so important? Consider what happens if you take your pills much earlier or later than you should or if you do not take them at all.

If you take your pills much too early or take more pills than you should, the amount of drug in your blood reaches much higher levels. Since higher levels are associated with increased side effects, you are more likely to experience undesirable symptoms caused by your medications. With the advances in new medicines, your doctor can make it easier for you to comply by using drugs which are effective and have few side effects, such as some ACE inhibitors, beta blockers, calcium channel blockers, and diuretics. By using long-acting agents, you need only one dose per day, which saves time and may save you money.

If you stop taking your pills altogether, your blood pressure may not only go back to the high levels recorded before you began treatment, it may "bounce back" even higher levels. The risk of this rebound hypertension is highest when using central agents such as Catapres (clonidine).

For these reasons, it is important that you never stop taking medication without consulting your doctor and that you follow the prescription for your medication as closely as possible. It is a good idea to learn the names of your medications and to bring your pill bottles to your doctor so that he or she is certain of which pills you are taking. You might consider noting the names and doses of your medication and keeping this information in your wallet or purse. Sometimes there is miscommunication between the doctor, patient, and/or pharmacist.

HANDY REMINDERS

These are some tips on how to remember to take your medications:

- Take the pills or capsules when you do some other routine task, such as brushing your teeth.

- Keep the pills in separate containers that are labeled with the time when you should take them, such as at breakfast, lunch, dinner, or at bedtime.
- Wear a watch with an alarm set for the times you need to take your medicines.
- Mark down on a calendar every time you take your medicine.
- At the beginning of each day, set out the pills that you need to take.
- Ask a family member or roommate to remind you to take your medication until you begin to remember on your own.
- Always make sure that you keep some extra pills in case you run out before the next visit to the doctor.
- Count your pills at the beginning and at the end of the week to see if you forgot to take any.

MEDICATION COSTS

About one in ten people with high blood pressure will need to take three or more different types of medicines in order to control their blood pressure. About one out of every one hundred patients will even require five or six different types! The costs of multiple medications can be a major problem. Ask the pharmacist in advance how much each drug will cost. It is useful to shop around for the best price; you could save as much as 50 percent. There is usually a savings if you can buy your medicines in quantities of fifty or one hundred rather than thirty. If you are age fifty-five or more, ask if there are special discounts available. Chapter 15 offers other tips to save you money on your blood pressure treatment.

GENERIC DRUGS

Tell your doctor if you are having problems with the medication costs. Several blood pressure drugs are now available as "generics." This means that a drug, originally developed by one company, is now marketed competitively by other companies. Generic high blood pressure drugs are cheaper for the pharmacist, and this cost savings is usually passed along to the customer. The generics have not undergone the extensive testing done by the company that originally developed them, but they meet important standards of the Food and Drug Administration, such as the absorption from the stomach and intestines into the body and the availability in the body of the active forms of the drug.

Generic medications usually have a different shape and color than the parent drug tablet or capsule. Therefore, if you switch to a generic drug, read the label carefully to be sure that it is the same drug and that the dosage (5, 10, 25, 50, 80, or 100 mg [milligrams]) and the dosage intervals (once, twice, three, or four times a day) are otherwise identical to what you were taking before. The same generic medication may be manufactured by different companies; therefore, the shape and color of the same medication may be different.

SUMMARY

If you feel bad after you begin treatment, check with your doctor. Your symptoms could be caused by your drug, and lowering the dose or switching to another drug might eliminate the bad effects while still providing the blood pressure control.

14

The Benefits of Treatment

So why treat your high blood pressure? Effective treatment of high blood pressure increases your chance for a longer life; it helps decrease your risk of a stroke, kidney disease, and heart disease; it also reduces the possibility of being paralyzed, being hooked up to a kidney machine for several hours each week, or needing open heart surgery or kidney transplantation.

BLOOD PRESSURE STUDIES

The benefits of blood pressure treatment have been proven through earlier studies that were prospective and randomized. In this type of study, a large group of people have their blood pressure taken. Those with high blood pressure are randomly divided into two or more groups.

One group is called the control group; they are not put on medication but are observed or sometimes treated with general health measures or special diets. Their blood pressures are measured regularly, and they receive X-rays, EKGs, and lab tests. They frequently do better than persons who do not choose to be in a research study. Those who are in the other groups take medications and are called the treatment groups. They are also examined periodically by doctors and nurses and are given various blood and other tests.

Statisticians analyze the results of these periodic examinations. If one group (either a control or a treatment group) has more heart attacks or strokes than the other group, and if the differences are significant, then the results are published in medical journals that provide continuing medical education for physicians in the community.

Such studies are called clinical trials and are approved and funded by panels of experts in the scientific review branches of the government or private industry. It is necessary to conduct such studies because when a single patient takes a drug and his health improves, it does not prove that all patients will also do as well. Some may, and some may not. However, we can know the odds fairly well by looking at the data from separate groups of patients.

THE VALUE OF HIGH BLOOD
PRESSURE MEDICINES

One of the first studies that clearly documented the value of taking blood pressure medication was the Veterans Administration Cooperative Study. In this study, conducted in the mid 1960s, many VA hospitals across the country enlisted large numbers of men with high blood pressure. Half of these men were given a combination pill with three different medications combined in one. The medications were a diuretic, reserpine, and hydralazine. The other group of men were not given any medications. The benefits of treatment were clear: fewer complications and fewer deaths.

Treatment of Moderate High Blood Pressure

One-third of the group of men with a diastolic (bottom number) blood pressure at 115 mm Hg or greater who were not on medication developed serious problems with their kidneys, heart, or brain. Two patients even died. Of those who did take medications, less than 10 percent experienced complications. There were no deaths among the treated patients.

About eleven months after the beginning of the study, these findings were noted and this part of the research was stopped. Then, all of the patients with an initial diastolic blood pressure equal to or greater than 115 mm Hg were started on medication. It took a little more than twenty months to determine that there were also major differences in the amount and severity of complications among those patients whose initial diastolic blood pressure was equal to or greater than 104 mm Hg and who were treated with drugs compared with those who were not. There were not enough people in the study to determine if drug treatment was appropriate at levels below 105 mm Hg (mild hypertension).

Treatment of Mild High Blood Pressure

The question then was: Should milder levels of diastolic high blood pressure (90-104 mm Hg) be treated with medication? To answer this, a multi-million-dollar study, The Hypertension Detection and Follow-up Program [HDFP], funded between 1973 and 1979 by the National Institutes of Health, was conducted at fourteen medical centers in the United States. The study also sought to determine if a major community-based effort to control high blood pressure could reduce the number of deaths from this disease.

At the start of the study, approximately 150,000 Americans were screened for high blood pressure at their home or workplace. Those with a diastolic blood pressure of 95 mm Hg or higher were referred to clinics. Then, of those whose repeat blood pressure was 90 mm Hg or greater, half were treated in clinics to try to reduce their blood pressure either to below 90 mm Hg or to 10 mm Hg below their initial blood pressure, whichever was lower. The other half were referred to their private doctors or community sources for treatment.

The results showed that those hypertensive patients who were treated regularly and had their blood pressures reduced the most had a much lower risk of stroke or death. This was true for patients with mild as well as moderate and severe high blood pressure.

In other words, it appeared that the very concerted effort to lower blood pressure resulted in fewer deaths. However, since there are many other studies that have looked at these issues, and the results sometimes conflict, there are questions that still remain about precisely how low of a level of mild high blood pressure should be treated with medication. As a result, doctors often decide on a patient-by-patient basis. For example, if your mother or father had high blood pressure or a stroke, if you already have a kidney problem or enlarged heart from high blood pressure, if you are black, or if you have other heart risk factors, then your doctor would probably start treating you with medication, even at the lowest range of high blood pressure.

Treatment of Systolic High Blood Pressure Alone

Many other persons may have a form of high blood pressure in which only the systolic (top number) is above normal (e.g., greater than 160 mm Hg) and the diastolic is normal (e.g., below 90 mm Hg). This is called isolated systolic hypertension. Whether treatment would result in benefit was not known until recently, although this type of high blood pressure is dangerous. A study called SHEP (Systolic Hypertension in the Elderly Program) was conducted in 16 medical centers around the country. Half of the subjects were treated with a diuretic or in combination with a beta blocker and half were not treated (control group). The results showed clear-cut benefit from treatment, resulting in a 36 percent reduction in strokes.

Treatment of High Blood Pressure Emergencies

While there have been controversies regarding the treatment of lower levels of high blood pressure, there has never been any doubt that the treatment of high blood pressure emergencies is lifesaving. As early as the 1950s, potent drugs (ganglionic blocking drugs) were given intravenously in a hospital when blood pressure was severely elevated and associated with brain, kidney, and sometimes heart damage. Patients' symptoms would include headaches, visual disturbances, and sometimes mental confusion or loss of consciousness. If treatment was not carried out promptly to lower their blood pressure, most of these patients would have died in a short period of time. Numerous studies and reports have shown that treatment will benefit such patients and prolong their lives considerably. In more recent years, newer drugs have become available that can control these emergency blood pressure situations with minimal hospital stay.

Continuing Debates

It is not surprising that at national or international meetings on high blood pressure, scientists, doctors, nurses, and other health providers still debate about which medicines to use, when to start treatment, how to evaluate the patients, and other related issues. These debates are very educational, and they remind us that we do not have all the answers. New discoveries continually change the issues, and perhaps, one day, a better understanding of what causes high blood pressure may enable us to develop a simple cure, such as a one-time shot or monthly pill that would make it easier for patients to keep their blood pressure under control.

Millions Benefit

In the meantime, the hundreds of millions of people in the world with high blood pressure are more fortunate than their ancestors. The chance of death from a stroke has been reduced by 50 percent in the United States since 1972 (Figure 6). The risk of death from a heart attack has been reduced more than 40 percent.

Today, patients can live normal, healthy lives by adhering to some simple preventive measures, such as losing weight, limiting dietary salt and cholesterol, quitting smoking, and if necessary, taking medications. There is a much greater choice of medications, and it is usually possible to select one that has a few side effects and works well. The results are better blood pressure control; less risk of stroke, heart attack, or kidney failure; and a longer and better quality of life.

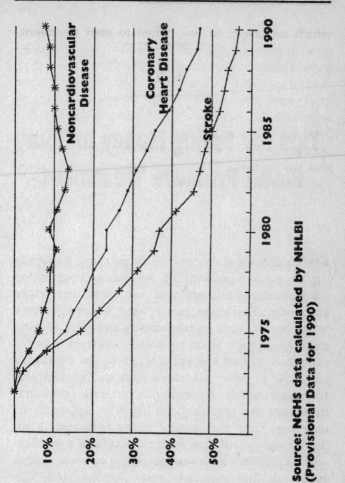

Figure 6. Percent Decline in Age-Adjusted Mortality Rates Since 1972

15

Tips for Saving Money In Your Blood Pressure Treatment

This chapter is written to help you save hundreds or even thousands of dollars on your blood pressure treatment and use your time more efficiently. There are many ways to save money when having your blood pressure treated. Learning more about high blood pressure makes you a better consumer so that you know when to see the doctor and how to better ask about tests and medications that are available. For example, ordering free literature from the organizations listed in Appendix III may save time and money in the long run. Also, don't forget to tell your doctor if you have a problem with expenses. He or she may know of some special assistance that may help you. The following tips may be helpful.

A. Blood Pressure Checks
1. Consider free blood pressure screenings or ask your doctor, dentist, or pharmacist if they would mind checking your blood pressure no matter what the reason for your visit.
2. Tests can often be obtained at screening programs, which you can find out about from your newspaper, the local Heart Association, Kidney Foundation, or hospital social worker. Show your findings to your doctor.
3. Record the time, day, and blood pressure levels on a list every time it is checked. Show your doctor so he or she has more recordings to use in assessing your condition.
4. Consider purchasing a blood pressure cuff at the drug store, a surgical supply house, or in a traditional discount department store. Blood pressure kits may also be available free of charge with some products. Ask your doctor when receiving the prescription. The cuff needs to be checked for accuracy regularly by comparing results to those recorded in your doctor's office. Also, make certain that you purchase the correct size cuff for the size of your arm. Your doctor may be willing to schedule your visits less frequently if you are monitoring your blood pressure as long as you notify him or her if the values change too much in one direction or the other, or if you develop symptoms or side effects. This could possibly save $50-$250 per year.

B. Medications
1. When starting new blood pressure medica-

tions, ask your doctor for free samples. This way, if you develop side effects or the medicine is not working well, you haven't spent $50-$100 on medicine you may not be able to use again.

2. Once you are on medication on a regular basis, you may wish to get the full supply at one time since there is often an additional charge for refills on each prescription.

3. Certain mail order programs such as those provided by the American Association of Retired Persons often provide medications at lower costs. However, personal services are often provided at the local pharmacy where you can ask about blood pressure medication side effects as well as reactions with other medicines.

4. Ask your doctor about special cost-saving programs and educational information provided by the manufacturer of blood pressure medications.

5. If you are indigent, your doctor may help you receive free medication by contacting the pharmaceutical manufacturer of your drug. Your doctor can get a list of these programs from the Pharmaceutical Manufacturer's Association in Washington, D.C., the International Society on Hypertension in Blacks in Atlanta, or the book entitled *Better Health Care for Less* (New York: Hippocrene).

6. Your doctor may refer you to the state health department if they provide services and treatment for blood pressure, or to a community health center that helps provide care at re-

duced cost for those who are in a financial bind. The National Association of Community Health Centers in Washington has lists of member centers and locations.

7. You or your doctor may wish to call the hypertension, cardiology, nephrology, or internal medicine department of a medical school to find out if any free studies are being conducted where you may save hundreds of dollars, since all medicines, tests, and visits are usually provided free.

8. You may wish to call different drugstores to compare prices of your medications. Remember, some drugstores may charge more for one pill and less for another. Recheck prices intermittently. You might also ask if the pharmacist will give you a discount, particularly if you know the competition has a lower price.

C. Doctor Visits
1. Some doctors arrange for nurses or physician's assistants to treat your blood pressure at a lower cost than the regular doctor's visit charge.

2. You should bring pill bottles and costs of medicines to your doctor so he or she can be more informed of your expenses.

3. You may ask your doctor to write prescriptions for a longer period of time if he or she thinks it is appropriate (for example, a six-month versus a three-month supply).

D. Laboratory and Other Tests
1. Always ask for copies of your lab, EKG, and chest X-ray results as well as other test results, keeping these on file at home so that you can

show them to referring doctors or doctors in emergency situations. This can save money by not having to order repeat tests. It may also improve the quality of your care by providing comparisons with earlier test results.

E. Hospitalizations for emergency blood pressure treatment or more sophisticated testing to evaluate for special causes of high blood pressure

1. For non-emergency admissions, attempt to request admission during the weekdays when the tests are usually performed, with proper scheduling of the tests in advance. This can eliminate extra days in the hospital.

2. Obtain pre-admission certification from your insurance carrier to make certain that they will give you maximum coverage.

3. If you are going to have difficulty paying your hospital bill, ask to see the hospital social worker on your first day of admission. You may be eligible for financial assistance.

4. Emergency treatment in the hospital emergency room is often covered with no deductible charged to you if the records indicate it is truly an emergency room visit.

5. Keep records in the hospital of all tests performed and medications received so you can verify the accuracy of your hospital bill on discharge.

6. Bring personal items (toothbrush, combs, etc.) to the hospital, for often they are more expensive if provided by the hospital.

7. Attempt to request hospital checkout prior to "discharge time" to save an extra day's charge (such as in a hotel).

8. Review your hospital bill closely and ask your doctor to glance at it and to point out any errors in "big ticket" items.

9. If you can't afford payment for your entire hospital stay, work out a payment schedule with the business office. The hospital usually won't charge interest.

10. Sometimes your doctor can arrange home health services so you can leave the hospital early and receive assistance from medical personnel even if bedridden.

F. Prevention is the biggest saving.

1. Taking your blood pressure medications regularly and taking proper preventive measures (reducing weight when appropriate, decreasing salt intake, and avoiding excess alcohol intake) can help save lots of money. Preventive measures may help reduce the amount of medicines you need to take. In addition, blood pressure control can reduce the risk of costly treatments for stroke, heart failure, heart attacks, vision problems, and kidney disease.

G. For a more comprehensive book on health care savings, consider reading the book *Better Health Care for Less*, by N.B. Shulman and L.S. Sweitzer (New York: Hippocrene).

Appendix I

High Blood Pressure Drug Directory*

LEGEND: CLASS OF DRUGS (SEE CHAPTER 9)

1 = Diuretic; 1ª = K-sparing
2 = Beta Blocker
3 = Calcium Channel Blocker
4 = ACE Inhibitor
5 = Alpha Blocker
6 = Central Agent
7 = Vasodilator
8 = HBP drug + a Diuretic
9 = Other

Accupril (quinapril)[4]
Adalat (nifedipine)[3]
Aldactazide[1a]
Aldactone (spironolactone)[1a]
Aldochlor[8] (class 1 + 6)
Aldomet (methyldopa)[6]
Aldoril[8] (class 1 + 6)
Altace (ramipril)[4]
Anhydron (cyclothiazide)[1]
Apresoline (hydralazine)[7]

Blocadren (timolol)[2]
Breviblok (esmolol)[2]

Bumex (bumetanide)[1]

Calan (verapamil)[3]
Calan SR[3]
Capoten (captopril)[4]
Capozide[8] (class 1 + 4)
Cardene (nicardipine)[3]
Cardene SR (nicardipine)[3]
Cardizem (diltiazem)[3]
Cardizem SR[3]
Cardura (doxazosin)[5]
Cartrol (carteolol)[2]
Catapres (clonidine)[6]
Catapres TTS Patch[6]

Combipres[8] (class 1 + 4)
Corgard (nadolol)[2]
Corzide[8] (class 1 + 2)

Diamox (acetazolamide)[1]
Dibenzyline (phenoxy-
   enzamine)[5]
Dilacor XR (diltiazem)[3]
Diucardin
   (hydroflumethiazide)[1]
Diulo (metolazone)[1]
Diuril (chlorothiazide)[1]
Dyazide[1a]
DynaCirc (isradipine)[3]
Dyrenium (triamterene)[1a]

Edecrin (ethacrinic acid)[1]
Enduron (methyclothiazide)[1]
Esidrix (hydrochlorothiazide)[1]
Exna (benzthiazide)[1]

Hydrochlorothiazide[1]
Hydromox (quinethazone)[1]
Hygroton (chlorthalidone)[1]
Hylorel (guanadrel)[9]
Hytrin (terazosin)[5]

Inderal (propranolol)[2]
Inderal LA[2]
Inderide[8] (class 1 + 2)
Ismelin (guanethidine)[9]
Isoptin (verapamil)[3]
Isoptin SR[3]

Kerlone (betaxolol)[2]

Lasix (furosemide)[1]
Levatol (penbutolol)[2]
Loniten (minoxidil)[7]
Lopressor (metoprolol)[2]
Lotensin (benazepril)[4]
Lozol (indapamide)[1]

Maxzide[1a]
Midamor (amiloride)[1a]
Minipress (prazosin)[5]
Minipress XL[5]
Moduretic[1a]
Monopril (fosinopril)[4]

Naqua (trichlormethiazide)[1]
Naturetin (bendroflume-
   thiazide)[1]
Nimotop (nimodipine)[3]
Normodyne (labetalol)[2,5]
Norvasc (amlodipine)[3]

Plendil (felodipine)[3]
Prazosin XL[5]
Procardia (nifedipine)[3]
Procardia XL[3]
Prinivil (lisinopril)[4]
Prinzide[8] (class 1 + 4)

Regitine (phentolamine)[5]
Renese (polythiazide)[1]
Reserpine[9]

Saluron (hydroflumethiazide)[1]
Sectral (acebutalol)[2]
Ser-Ap-Es[9]

Tenex (guanfacine)[6]

Tenormin (atenolol)[2]
Tenoretic[8] (class 1 + 2)
Toprol XL (metoprolol)[2]
Trandate (labetalol)[2,5]

Vascor (bepridil)[3]
Vasoretic[8] (class 1 + 4)
Vasotec (enalapril)[4]
Verelan (verapamil)[3]

Visken (pindolol)[2]

Wytensin (guanabenz)[6]

Zaroxolyn (metolazone)[1]
Zebeta (bisoprolol)[2]
Zestoretic[8] (class 1 + 4)
Zestril (lisinopril)[4]

*There are hundreds of high blood pressure drugs available, and all are not listed here, but included are examples of all of the types. The capitalized name is the trade, brand, or company name of the drug, whereas the name in parentheses is the generic name of the drug. The numbers in the legend refer to the type of drug.

Appendix II

Additional Reading on High Blood Pressure

American Heart Association Diet, copies available (1 copy free, 100 copies for $10.70) from the American Heart Association, 1615 Stemmons Freeway, Dallas, TX 75207-8806.

Better Health Care for Less, by N.B. Shulman, M.D. and L.S. Sweitzer, M.D., New York: Hippocrene, 1992.

Cardiovascular Diseases and Stroke in African-Americans and Other Racial Minorities in the United States, the American Heart Association, 1991 (professional reading).

Cardiovascular Diseases in Blacks, by E. Saunders, M.D., Philadelphia: F.A. Davis Company, 1991 (professional reading).

Clinical Hypertension, 5th Edition, by N.M. Kaplan, M.D., Baltimore: Williams & Wilkins, 1990 (professional reading).

Community Prevention and Control of Cardiovascular Diseases, World Health Organization, Technical Report Series 732, 1986. Copies can be purchased for U.S. $4.50 or for 9 Sw. Fr. from either WHO, Publication Center, 49 Sheridan Avenue, Albany NY 12210, or WHO, Distribution and Sales Service, 1211 Geneva 27, Switzerland.

Cooking Without Your Salt Shaker, Copies available for $4.50 from the American Heart Association, 7320 Greenville Avenue, Dallas, TX 75231.

Food Values of Portions Commonly Used, by J.A.T. Pennington, Ph.D., and H.N. Church, B.S., Philadelphia: J.P. Lippincott Company, 1980.

Hypertension in Blacks: Epidemiology, Pathophysiology and Treatment, by W.D. Hall, M.D., E. Saunders, M.D., and N.B. Shulman, M.D., Chicago: Year Book Medical Publishers, Inc., 1985 (professional reading).

Management of Arterial Hypertension: A Practical Guide for the Physician and Allied Health Workers, World Health Organization, 1985. (See Community Prevention for WHO addresses.)

Managing Hypertension: The Complete Program Developed by the Cleveland Clinic, by J.V. Warren, M.D. and G.J. Subak-Sharp, Garden City, NY: Doubleday & Company, Inc., 1986.

National Consensus Statement on Non-Pharmacological Therapy, Nonpharmacological Approaches to the Control of High Blood Pressure. Final Report of the Subcommittee on Detection, Evaluation, and Treatment of High Blood Pressure. Published in the medical journal *Hypertension*, volume 8, number 5, pages 444-467, May 1986. (The article contains 248 references.)

The Sodium Content of Your Food, U.S. Department of Agriculture, House and Garden Bulletin No. 223, 43 pages. Copies available for $2.25 from Superintendent of Documents, U.S. Government Printing Office, Washington, DC 20402.

Appendix III

Additional Resources for High Blood Pressure Information

There are numerous private organizations and governmental agencies to which you can write for information on high blood pressure detection, diet, weight reduction, and how to stay on therapy, and to find out where you might go for an educational program or have your blood pressure measured as part of a blood pressure screening program. We have listed many of these below.

You can also ask your physician, local health department, heart association, hospital staff, dietitian, dentist, or podiatrist whether they have such information. Your pharmacist may also be a good source of information, since many of the pharmaceutical companies offer booklets on this subject.

As you build your own understanding of high blood pressure and learn the importance of controlling this condition, you may find you would like to help others do this as well. Most of the service organizations rely heavily on volunteers and would welcome your help. We encourage you to find out which organizations have local chapters in your area and, if you can, to become active in their work. Helping others is one of the best ways to help yourself.

First and foremost, stay informed, check with your doctor on a regular basis, and follow your prescribed treatment plan. The result will be a longer and healthier life. We have seen this in so many of our patients, and we encourage you to claim these benefits for yourself.

UNITED STATES

National High Blood Pressure Education Program

This is a nationwide program to increase the detection and control of high blood pressure. The staff can provide you with printed information on high blood pressure for patients, consumers, and health professionals, and refer you to appropriate organizations for blood pressure screening programs and for developing community programs. Write:

National Blood Pressure Information Center
120/80 National Institutes of Health
Bethesda, MD 20892
301-951-3260

Public Health Departments

To find what resources are available in public health programs in your area, contact your state and local public health departments. High blood pressure programs may be included under their programs for chronic diseases, cardiovascular diseases, or hypertension.

American Heart Association

The Heart Association has long been active in programs to control high blood pressure. For printed materials and information on education and screening programs, contact your local chapter or write to the national clearinghouse:

American Heart Association
Office of Communications
1615 Stemmons Freeway
Dallas, TX 75207-8806
214-748-7212

International Society on Hypertension in Blacks (ISHIB)

ISHIB is focused on providing literature for patients, lists of special programs for those who cannot afford medication, scientific journals on diseases by ethnic groups, international conferences, and a heart-to-heart program to bring children from developing countries to the U.S. for free heart surgery. Contact:

International Society on Hypertension in Blacks
69 Butler Street, S.E.
Atlanta, GA 30303
404-616-3810

American Lung Association

The Lung Association provides information on how to stop smoking. Contact the local chapter in the nearest major city or the national office:

American Lung Association
1740 Broadway
New York, NY 10019
212-315-8700

National Kidney Foundation

This organization provides information on kidney disease and blood pressure. Contact the local chapter in the nearest major city or the national office:

National Kidney Foundation
30 East 33rd Street
New York, NY 10016
212-889-2210

Red Cross

Many chapters of the American Red Cross offer courses on blood pressure control and conduct blood pressure screenings. Contact your local chapter for the brochure, "The Lowdown on High Blood Pressure," and for information such as the dates and locations of health fairs where you can have your blood pressure checked. The national offices are in Washington, DC:

American Red Cross
430 17th Street, N.W.
Washington, DC 20006
202-737-8300

U.S. Pharmacopoeial Convention, Inc.

This nonprofit organization publishes, "About Your High Blood Pressure Medicines," which describes in understandable language the various high blood pressure medications and their possible unwanted side effects. To order this publication, send your name and address with a check or money order for $7.50 to:

U.S.P.C., Inc.
12601 Twin Brook Parkway
Rockville, MD 20852
301-881-0666

CANADA

Public Health

To find what resources are available in your area for public health programs and consumer information, contact your provincial Ministry of Health, which is listed in the special governmental section of the telephone directory.

Canadian Heart Foundation

This organization provides printed material on high blood pressure and conducts blood pressure screening and educational programs. Contact the Heart and Stroke Foundation Office in your province, or contact the national office:

Canadian Heart Foundation
160 George Street, Suite 200
Ottawa, Ontario K1N M2
613-237-4361

Canadian Lung Association

This organization provides literature and "countdown" programs to help you stop smoking. For information on what is offered by the provincial chapters, contact the national office:

Canadian Lung Association
1900 City Park Drive, Suite 508
Gloucester, Ontario K1J 1A3
613-747-6776

Kidney Foundation of Canada

This foundation provides information on high blood pressure and conducts screening programs. There are branches of the foundation in each province, usually in the capital city. For further information, contact the national office:

Kidney Foundation of Canada
6767 Cote des Neiges, Suite 301
Montreal, Quebec H3S 2T6
514-341-5422

INTERNATIONAL

World Health Organization

This organization can help you to identify blood pressure campaigns in various countries around the world. They also publish "Community Prevention and Control of Cardiovascular Diseases," Technical Report Series 732, 1986, for governments and private citizens, which describes how to develop programs at the local level. This can be purchased for 9 Sw. Fr. or U.S. $4.50 fee from either:

WHO
Distribution and Sales Service
1211 Geneva 27
Switzerland
or:
WHO
Publication Center
49 Sheridan Avenue
Albany, NY 12210
518-436-9686

Red Cross

The Red Cross offers information on high blood pressure and conducts blood pressure screenings in most countries. Contact the office in your capital city, or write the international headquarters:

International Red Cross
P.O. Box 372
CH 1211
Geneva 19
Switzerland
Telephone: 41 22 345580

Public Health Programs

Many countries conduct high blood pressure information and screening programs. To find what is available in your country, contact your government's Department or Ministry of Health.

Heart Foundation

National heart foundations have been organized in many countries. The main office is usually located in the capital or the largest city and often can supply printed materials, and information on blood pressure screenings and educational programs.

Glossary

High Blood Pressure
Patient's Dictionary

ACE inhibitors drugs like Capoten or Vasotec that
slow down the production of angiotensin converting enzyme (ACE). This keeps the body
from making angiotensin II, a powerful hormone that squeezes blood vessels and causes
blood pressure to rise.

albuminuria the presence of the protein albumin in
the urine. This usually indicates some problem
with the kidneys, such as nephritis or high
blood pressure.

aldosterone a hormone made by the adrenal gland.
It causes the kidneys to retain salt and raise
blood pressure.

aldosteronoma a small and usually noncancerous abnormal growth in the adrenal gland that makes
the hormone aldosterone and can cause high
blood pressure.

alpha blocker a drug that blocks tiny nerve fibers called alpha receptors. Examples of alpha blockers are Cardura, Hytrin, and Minipress.

aneurysm distension or ballooning of an artery, usually in the brain, aorta, or abdomen.

angina a chest discomfort or tightness, usually under the breastbone, that comes on with exertion and is relieved by rest. It may mean poor blood supply to the heart.

angioplasty blowing up a tiny balloon within the narrow part of an artery to make it wider.

aorta the main blood vessel (artery) of the body, originating from the heart.

arrhythmia an irregular heartbeat.

arteries blood vessels that carry blood to a tissue or organ of the body. Veins carry blood away from the tissue or organ. Red blood spurts from arteries; dark blood drips from vein.

arteriosclerosis hardening of the arteries.

beta blocker a high blood pressure drug that blocks the action of adrenaline on "beta" receptors in the body and tends to slow the heart rate. Examples include Blocadren, Corgard, Inderal, Kerlone, Levacor, Timolol, and Visken.

blood pressure the pressure or tension of the blood inside the arteries.

bradycardia a slow heartbeat, usually less than fifty to fifty-five times a minute.

bruit a noise over an artery that means it might be narrowed. Heard with a stethoscope. It can sometimes be heard over the neck (carotid bruit), abdomen (abdominal bruit), or groin (femoral bruit).

BUN blood urea nitrogen. A waste product that is formed from proteins and measured in the bloodstream. Normal is 5 to 20 mg/dl (milligrams per deciliter).

calcium a chemical (Ca) in the body that is necessary for muscles to squeeze down and for certain structures (bone, teeth, nails) to remain firm.

calcium channel blocker a high blood pressure drug that blocks calcium channels in body cells, keeping calcium out of the cell so that it can't contract as hard.

cardiomegaly an enlarged heart.

cardiovascular relating to the heart and blood vessels.

casts tiny "look-alikes" of parts of the kidney pipes found in the urine. They may be seen under a microscope and indicate kidney problems.

CAT scan see *scan.*

catecholamines blood hormones that can make you feel tense and nervous. They include epinephrine (commonly called adrenaline), norepinephrine, and dopamine.

CBC complete blood count. This blood test helps tell if there is any anemia or infection.

central agents blood pressure drugs that act mainly on the brain. Examples include Aldomet, Catapres, Tenex, and Wytensin.

cerebrovascular accident (CVA) a stroke.

cholesterol one of the fats in the blood that causes hardening of the arteries. A good cholesterol level in the blood is less than 200 mg/dl; 170 mg/dl is even better.

claudication severe cramps in the calves of the legs

or hips that come on during walking and are relieved by rest; caused by poor blood supply to the legs.

coarctation a marked narrowing of the main blood vessel of the body, the aorta, causing high blood pressure, particularly in children. Can be cured by surgery.

compliance doing what you are supposed to about your diet, medicines, and doctor's appointments in response to your high blood pressure.

congestive heart failure (CHF) when the heart becomes so weak that it fails and causes congestion in the lungs. See also _heart failure_.

constriction a clamping-down, squeezing, or narrowing.

coronary arteries the three blood vessels (arteries) that supply blood from the main blood vessel (aorta) to the heart.

coronary heart disease when the heart does not get enough nourishment from the blood vessels that feed it (that is, the coronary arteries). Symptoms include angina or heart attack.

creatinine a blood test that shows how well your kidneys are able to filter out things you don't need. Normal is 0.5 to 1.3 mg/dl.

Cushing's syndrome when high blood pressure is caused by too much of the hormone cortisol, made by the adrenal gland. Patients usually bruise easily and gain weight in their stomach and face.

dialysis the filtering out, by machine, of poisons that the kidneys can't get rid of when they are damaged or stop functioning.

diastolic   the bottom number of the blood pressure reading; the pressure in the arteries when the heart is relaxed.

diastolic hypertension   the diagnosis when the diastolic pressure (bottom number) is at least 90 mm Hg on several consecutive occasions.

diuretics   blood pressure medicines that cause your kidneys to get rid of extra salt and water. Examples include hydrochlorothiazide, HydroDIURIL, Hygroton, Lozol, Naqua, Naturetin and Zaroxolyn.

DSA   Digital Subtraction Angiogram. A special computerized X-ray of your kidneys to show whether there is narrowing of the artery that supplies blood to the kidneys.

dyspnea   shortness of breath.

ECHO   see *echocardiogram*.

echocardiogram   a painless test that bounces sound waves off your heart and takes pictures to see how thick the walls and how wide the chambers are.

eclampsia   when convulsions (seizures, epilepsy) occur in a pregnant woman with preeclampsia. See *preeclampsia*.

edema   a collection of fluid, or swelling, usually of the feet and eyes.

EKG/ECG   see *electrocardiogram*.

electrocardiogram   a painless test that records the electrical impulses from your heart onto a long strip of paper.

electrolytes   chemicals in the blood, usually including sodium (Na), potassium (K), chloride (Cl), and bicarbonate (HCO_3).

epinephrine   one of the hormones (catecholamines) made by the adrenal gland just above the kidney.

essential hypertension the most common type of high blood pressure, where the cause is unknown. Also called "primary" hypertension.

eyegrounds the arteries, veins, nerves, and the background of the eye that can be seen directly by looking in the eye with a light.

family history whether or not your parents, brothers, sisters, or their relatives had certain diseases such as high blood pressure or diabetes. High blood pressure tends to run in families.

fundi see _eyegrounds_.

gallop a sound that can be heard over your heart if it is straining too much to pump the blood out.

generic the general or primary name of a drug.

glucose a type of carbohydrate fuel in the blood that helps nourish body tissues. See also _sugar._

gout a very painful type of arthritis, usually associated with swelling and redness of the toe or foot. Caused by sharp needle-like crystals (uric acid) that come out of the blood and stick the joint.

gynecomastia a swelling of one or both breasts in men or women, which usually occurs just beneath and around the nipple and may be tender.

HDL High Density Lipoprotein. A "good guy" type of fat in the blood that eats up the "bad guys" (cholesterol, triglycerides). Unlike cholesterol, a high level of HDL (60 to 80 mg/dl) is good, and a low level (20 to 35 mg/dl) is bad.

heart failure when the heart can't pump well anymore and water accumulates in the lungs (water on the lungs) or legs (edema), causing shortness of breath. Called dropsy in the old days. Often abbreviated as CHF, or congestive heart failure.

hematocrit the portion of your blood that is made up by red blood cells. Normal is 38 to 45 volumes percent (vol %).

hemoglobin a protein in red blood cells that carries oxygen to the tissues. Normal is 12.5 to 15 vol %.

Holter monitor a special heart test done by attaching a patient to a battery and wires to check his or her EKG for a twenty-four-hour period of time. It helps pick up skippy beats and other irregularities of the heart.

hormones substances made by the glands in the body that affect specific tissues. Examples include thyroid hormone made by the thyroid gland, estrogens made by the ovary, and cortisol, aldosterone, or epinephrine made by the adrenal gland.

hypertension high blood pressure. When the diastolic blood pressure consistently exceeds 90 mm Hg or the systolic blood pressure exceeds 160. See *systolic* and *diastolic*.

hypokalemia a condition that develops when the blood level of serum potassium is too low, below 3.5 mEq/L.

impotence loss of sexual desire, loss of sexual ability, or inability to obtain/maintain erection.

ischemia when the blood supply to a tissue is less than what it needs. In the brain, ischemia can lead to stroke; in the heart, it can lead to a heart attack; in the legs, it can cause claudication or gangrene.

isolated systolic hypertension when the systolic pressure (top number) is 160 mm Hg or more but the diastolic pressure (bottom number) is below 90.

IVP Intravenous Pyelogram. An X-ray where dye is put into your arm and photographs of your kidneys and bladder are made for the next thirty to forty-five minutes.

lipids fats in the blood, including cholesterol and triglycerides.

LVH Left Ventricular Hypertrophy. When the muscle on the main (left) side of your heart has enlarged in order to handle the extra pressure put on it by high blood pressure.

magnesium a chemical (Mg) in the body that helps muscles and nerves to function normally.

malignant hypertension a condition where severe high blood pressure causes papilledema, a swelling of the nerve that goes to the eye. It is called malignant because, before good drug therapies were available, patients had a poor survival rate, much like patients with malignant cancers.

metanephrine a breakdown product of catecholamines that can be measured in the urine as a screening test to rule out a pheochromocytoma.

mitral valve prolapse when one of the main valves (mitral) on the left side of the heart has a floppy portion that makes a murmur and a clicky sound.

murmur a sound that may be heard over the heart with a stethoscope caused by blood flowing through a valve of the heart.

myocardial infarction heart attack; death of part of the heart muscle.

norepinephrine one of the hormones (catecholamines) that is made by the nerves of the body.

obesity usually when your body weight is 15 percent more than it should be for your height. For example, if you weigh 138 and should weigh 120, your body weight would be at 115 percent.

ophthalmoscope   the piece of equipment and light used by the doctor to look into our eyes.

orthostatic hypotension   sudden low blood pressure when you stand up.

over-the-counter   medications you can get at a drugstore without a prescription; sometimes also called patent medicines.

palpitations   pounding or skippy heart beats; "flip-flops."

papilledema   a swelling of the optic nerve that enters the back of the eye.

paresthesias   unusual tingly or crawly sensations, usually in the arms or legs.

pheochromocytoma   a tumor of the tiny adrenal gland just over the kidneys. It can release hormones that cause sudden high blood pressure, racing heart, sweating, and nervousness.

plaque   a buildup of fats (cholesterol, triglycerides) and other substances on the inside of an artery, making it narrower.

potassium   a mineral (K) in the body that is necessary for muscles to contract and nerves to fire. It gives strength to muscles. It often gets "washed out" by diuretics.

potassium-sparing diuretics   water pills that cause the kidneys to retain, rather than lose, potassium.

preeclampsia   a high blood pressure condition that can occur in the last few months of pregnancy.

primary hypertension   see *essential hypertension.*

proteinuria   the presence of protein in the urine,

which usually reflects some problem with the kidneys. See also *albuminuria*.

renal   pertaining to the kidneys.

renal artery stenosis   a narrowing (stenosis) of one or more of the renal arteries, which supply blood to the kidneys.

renin   an enzyme made by the kidneys. It can cause high blood pressure if there is too much of it.

renovascular hypertension   high blood pressure resulting from renal artery stenosis (see above).

salt   NaCl, a crystallized form of sodium (Na) plus chloride (Cl). One teaspoon contains 5 grams of salt = 2 grams of sodium = 70 milliequivalents of sodium.

salt substitutes   products that look like salt but taste somewhat more bitter because they contain potassium chloride. Usually used to reduce the amount of salt or increase the amount of potassium in your diet.

scan   a test in which you are given a small amount of a radioactive substance and machines determine where it travels by how many ticks it gives off. A computerized axial tomography (CAT) scan usually involves no injection of a radioactive substance.

secondary hypertension   high blood pressure that is secondary to a specific cause, such as renal artery stenosis.

sediment   the part of urine that can be examined under a microscope after it has been separated in a centrifuge.

side effect   an adverse or bad effect, usually of a drug.

skippy beats when your heart misses a beat, flutters, or "flip-flops."

sodium a mineral (Na) in the body that is necessary to help keep fluids distributed. It is the "Na" part of salt (NaCl).

sphygmomanometer a machine used to measure blood pressure.

stenosis a narrowing.

stethoscope an instrument used by a clinician to listen for sounds over your heart or other parts of your body.

stroke when parts of the brain are so low in blood supply that they stop working and cause paralysis of an arm and leg or inability to talk straight or problems with vision. See also *ischemia*.

sugar in medicine, sugar usually means glucose. Glucose is formed in the body from carbohydrates in the diet. Too much glucose in the blood is diabetes; thus, diabetic patients are sometimes said to have "sugar."

syncope a sudden and usually temporary loss of consciousness, such as fainting.

systolic the top number of the blood pressure reading; the pressure in the arteries when the heart is pumping.

tachycardia a rapid heartbeat, usually over one hundred times a minute.

target organs the organs of the body that are most adversely affected by untreated high blood pressure. These include primarily the heart, brain, kidneys, and eyes.

thiazide diuretic a commonly prescribed type of water pill (diuretic).

thrombosis   a clot that partially or completely blocks a blood vessel, such as coronary artery thrombosis or cerebral artery thrombosis.

TIA   Transient Ischemic Attack. A "near stroke" that occurs when parts of the brain don't get enough blood and a part of the body loses function for a few minutes.

toxemia   a toxic state of high blood pressure that can occur in the last few months of pregnancy. Also called preeclampsia.

trade name   the brand name of a drug as made by a specific company.

triglycerides   one of the types of fat in the blood.

ultrasound   a special painless X-ray test that bounces sound waves off parts of your body (e.g., the kidneys) to tell how big the organ is and whether the texture is soft or hard.

uremia   a condition in which the kidneys can no longer get rid of poisons that have accumulated in the blood, causing you to lose your appetite, become nauseated, and generally feel terrible.

uric acid   a chemical in the blood that can cause gout if its level gets too high and its sharp crystals are filtered out of the bloodstream and embedded in a joint.

vasoconstriction   when the blood vessels squeeze and clamp down.

vasodilator   a type of blood pressure drug that directly relaxes the blood vessels. Examples include Apresoline and Loniten.

water pills   see *diuretics*.

Index